3 Off the Tee:

NO EXCUSES

THE **FIT MIND-FIT BODY**

STRATEGY BOOK

Lorii Myers

3 Off the Tee: **No Excuses**
The Fit Mind-Fit Body Strategy Book
by Lorii Myers

i Leda Publishing Corp.

667 Welham Road, Suite 5
Barrie, ON, Canada L4N-0B7

ISBN-10: 0986790079
EAN-13: 9780986790072

Unattributed quotations by Lorii Myers.

Author photograph by Nat Caron Photography.

No Excuses is the third in a series of motivational, self-improvement books to be published under the *3 Off the Tee* brand.

This book is dedicated to my daughter, Jill, and all who endeavor to fuel and protect their minds and bodies against the environment, the test of time, and unnecessary, unwarranted excuses.

Table of Contents

Preface

This year my mom and dad celebrate their seventieth wedding anniversary. My mom is in her early nineties, my dad in his late eighties, and they have lived long, full, happy, healthy lives. They have both had illnesses and setbacks in their later years: my dad has survived lymphoma and a broken hip and has endured a long battle with cancer, and my mom has struggled with osteoarthritis, high blood pressure, and an underactive thyroid. Yet they have both managed not only to live longer than their own parents, but to live engaged and active lives.

This leaves me with a steadfast and conscientious desire to do the same. I would be delighted to live to one hundred and fifty years of age as long as I am happy, healthy, and still have my wits about me.

Assuming that I may have another forty to fifty years of life ahead of me—and yes, I know there are no guarantees—I wholeheartedly commit to a no-excuses lifestyle, and I aspire to make possibilities become realities.

This is not a revelation for me. I committed to a mindful health regimen back in my college days when I struggled with my own body image. Back then, I was far too hard on myself. Over the years it has become blatantly clear to me that kindness and patience plays a big role in our ability to change and grow. Don't beat yourself up for your shortcomings; delight in the prospect of what you will do, what you will achieve, and who you will become.

This book is intended to teach you how to exercise your mind and body in a new way. If your mind and body are working in unison, you can achieve great things in your life. Your body will become strong and resilient, and as a result, you will feel confident, fit, and in control.

Your healthy body will fuel your brain and keep your mind sharp. You will be able to focus, adapt, and realign as required. You won't get lost or sidetracked by unimportant factors or excuses along the way.

Maintaining a healthy mind and body is life's greatest achievement. Reinforcing the connection of body, mind, and achievement is crucial to developing your mental acuity and physical stamina. Almost everything of importance that you tackle will require continued staying power—over the long haul, you have to stay the course.

The golf-as-life metaphor works like this: you play every day as if it's a new day. You approach your day by strategizing how to get the maximum impact for that day (the best shot, as it were). You need to set yourself up right, keep your head in the game, and keep an accurate score of how you are performing so you can plan for continual improvement as you move forward to your ultimate goal. This is the process of improvement—you live smart, you practice, you plan, you lower your score, and you succeed.

I believe we can all take control of our lives using mental and physical life strategies. I challenge you to read on and, ultimately, to prove me right!

Enough said—we have work to do!

Hit 'em straight,

Lorii

Lorii@3-Off-the-Tee.com

Introduction

Tee shot. Slice...yikes

Do I drop a ball or go three off the tee?

I regroup and reload.

I'm going for it.

Deep breath. Loose grip. Swing thought.

I'm in the zone...

When you're in this position, you always have a choice—

you have decisions to make.

Finally, I've got my game on. I'm trying not to think too hard about it, trying not to overthink my game—and then I slice the ball.

If you are not a golfer, let me take a minute to explain what a slice is. In golf, a tee shot is simply the first shot on a hole where the ball has been hit off a tee. You're at the tee box with good intentions of driving your ball straight down the fairway (the closely mowed area between the tee and the green). But sometimes, when you slice the ball off the tee, instead of going straight down the fairway, it curves wildly from left to right (for a right-handed player) and ultimately veers drastically to the right and away from your target.

You can slice deep into the bush, a sand trap, or even water, to name a few of the standard obstacles on a golf course. Sometimes the sliced ball is going to end up somewhere that you don't want it to be.

When this happens in recreational golf, Rule #27 from the rule book called *The Rules of Golf: Through 1999* (Tom Watson, Frank Hannigan, Pocket Books, 1999) kicks into play. It states that if you lose a ball hit from the tee, you can hit from the tee again or drop a ball two club lengths back from where your ball exited the fairway. Either way, your score is one stroke from the tee plus one penalty stroke for the lost ball. In other words, you are now hitting your third shot—one stroke for the lost shot plus the other two from the tee. Thus the term *three off the tee*.

Now let's apply the same kind of scenario to your life. Imagine for a moment that you have this thought: "I seem to be running in place. I'm sidetracking, moving forward and backward, but always ending up back in the same space."

Usually when something goes wrong in your life, like a slice in golf, you start thinking of all the bad things that could happen to you instead of how you're going to fix the problem. Rather than think of the negatives, this is when you need to pay attention and make decisions. Yet this is where most of us start to conjure up a story in our mind, one that will support the idea that whatever just happened is not our fault—in other words, "The Excuse."

Everyone faces challenges in their day-to-day lives. But the defining moments of how successful you may be in life, both personally and professionally, lie in how you work through the process of recognizing, navigating, and ultimately dealing with all the inevitable hazards that life throws in your path.

I love the game of golf, and I love it because, as in any game, you are always trying to improve. In golf, you're always working on your abilities and skills, but you also want to improve your score. And that's what makes golf a great metaphor for your life. In the everyday world, you want to get better at carving out a life that you enjoy, but you also want to improve your skill-sets and knowledge base so you are better able to see opportunities and chase them down—that's the "score" part.

Golf is also a great metaphor for your personal and business life because in golf, as in life, you are most often competing with yourself first, so you have to be honest with yourself and you have to be open to change and growth. You must always accept that the scorecard tells all, whether you are making progress or not, and it tells you where you need to focus.

Do you find yourself making excuses in order to explain why you are still doing what you have always done? Are you aware that this equates to running in place for the rest of your life? If you can admit to these two things, you'll find, as you work through this book that you'll be able to break through these barriers and take positive action more often than you may think.

In this book, I am going to walk you through a model that will help you identify and crush excuses. More than that, though, I am going to challenge you to work through this model with me to build a No Excuses Success Action Plan (SAP) and then create a working lifestyle prototype—a personalized program that focuses on infusing a succession of small, incremental positive changes into your life that in time will become automatic winning habits for you.

The three top goals people target yet fail to achieve concern fitness—losing weight, getting in shape, and becoming healthier overall—and these areas are where excuses build up, usually causing willpower to falter and failure to prevail. So this is where we are going to start. We are going to replace excuses with winning habits. Are you up for a no-excuses challenge coupled with a fitness challenge?

Before you answer, let me define *fitness* with respect to the context of this book. The definition is twofold. First, we are going to delve into what it takes to build an action plan—the No Excuses Success Action Plan (SAP)—for a fit mind, one that is resilient and durable, one that won't succumb to excuses. Second, we are going to force that action plan into play with solid working examples in chapters 10 through 18 and then explore what it takes to build a fit lifestyle, one that is healthful and strong and an expression of your inner confidence. The resulting lifestyle prototype will become your personal body brand. Consider the prospect of exercising your mind and body in a new way, in tandem, and reaping the benefits of the mind-body-achievement connection.

This is the lifestyle I live, and I achieved this level of fitness by being relentless about transforming myself into the best shape of my life by the nineteenth hole. There was no lip service—I worked through the nineteen holes presented in this book, and I achieved my fitness goals. And you can too.

If you're open and willing to learn how to set aside your excuses—great, let's go! If you need help to get psyched up, then put your protective headgear on and continue reading. We'll get ramped up together, building a game plan and an action plan.

By working through the model described in this book, you will not only get in shape, you will learn how to easily recognize, manage, and ultimately obliterate excuses—all excuses—not only those interfering with your fitness track. You will be armed and ready with solid visualization strategies geared toward success that, once incorporated into your day-to-day life, will support your No Excuses SAP and lifestyle.

As you read, you will find that you are either on the front nine, the turn, the back nine, or the nineteenth hole. I use a round of golf as the structure for my book series to offer a fresh, streamlined, and easy-to-use format, but it's also meant to reinforce a healthy, competitive mind–body connection and keep it ever-present throughout the books.

It is my objective to help you learn how to say no to day-to-day excuses so you can build an authentic lifestyle prototype that consists of a game plan to create a strong mind, a sleek physique, and optimal health. If you can take on and conquer this goal, one of the toughest challenges there is, there will be no stopping you in whatever you choose to tackle.

There are many life analogies in golf, and you're going to read about them in the pages that follow. But *3 Off the Tee: No Excuses* isn't just a golf book; it's your personal challenge to improve by removing excuses and taking a good hard look at what is important in your life. By using healthful competition, taking responsibility for what is good and bad in your life, planning for improvement, and taking hazards out of play, you can reinvent your world. In essence, we are going to focus on strategically replacing excuses with winning habits, which are the ultimate excuse blockers.

If you are reading this book, you already recognize the value of improving. You are working to improve yourself and make yourself more successful and effective. As you begin or progress in your journey in life, think about having a personal scorecard on which you can record how you're doing on a regular basis. Succeeding in life is so much easier when you take just this one step because, with that scorecard, you can focus on what is important for your goals, deal with day-to-day obstacles, and make good decisions.

What I hope you get out of this book is inspiration, direction, awareness, and confidence in grabbing hold of challenge, brainstorming, and coming up with ideas and solutions rather than excuses.

As you read, think of the following three sentences as your mantra:

o I thrive on seeking out new opportunities. Once I'm on board, the challenge is mine.

o I am not deterred when I make a bad play; I just regroup and keep on going.

o Ultimately, I know that a bad play simply means I still have some work to do.

Also, I want you to think about what *no excuses* means to you. Is it just a catch phrase, or is it how you truly want to live your life? Do you sometimes make excuses, taking the easy way out? Would you rather be motivated, challenged, and inspired?

The no-excuses attitude is a process. It doesn't happen overnight. It involves assessing where you are at present, knowing where you are heading, and making good decisions along the way. This book is about becoming limitless, your mind and body working in harmony and directed at achieving a targeted, successful outcome.

This book is really two books in one. The front nine section explains the No Excuses Success Action Plan, with components necessary to turn aspirations into expectations in both your personal and business life roles. The back nine section explains the resulting lifestyle prototype, which involves applying SAP to real-life challenges using specific examples. Specifically, the examples I am using will help to create a strong mind, sleek physique, and optimal health. It's a great way to familiarize yourself with the mind-body-achievement connection and how to use it to achieve personal success in your own life.

Now let me throw out a simple statement: *when you master my challenge on the back nine, you will have also developed the tools needed to turn your aspirations into expectations.* I hope this not only catches your attention but that you believe it. This is the first step on your path to a No Excuses lifestyle.

Ready? Tee up and let's go!

The Front Nine:
The Success Action Plan (SAP)

Course Management

The 1st Hole – Be Limitless
The 2nd Hole – The Aerial Perspective
The 3rd Hole – Aspirations
The 4th Hole – Excuse Management
The 5th Hole – The BIG Push
The 6th Hole – Motivation
The 7th Hole – Inspiration and Incentive
The 8th Hole – The Vision
The 9th Hole – Master Strategy

The quest of any game in its simplest form—to be the best you can be and work toward making the win.

If there is one overriding principle in golf, it is the principle of course management. There's a lot to consider, such as knowing the problems or hazards of the course and how to cope with them in order to score consistently. You have to play smart and position your shots so you can place the ball in the "A" position—that position that allows the best approach for your next shot. Every play counts.

I have spent a great deal of time considering the value of course management in golf. It begins with knowing the layout of the course hole by hole. You rationalize your best shot by mentally playing each hole forward and in reverse: from the tee to the green, and from the green to the tee.

The value of having a vision and the ability to strategize and focus is probably so obvious that I have you thinking, "Lorii, you're preaching to the choir!" But hear me out. The habits developed from using good course management force you to think clearly before taking every shot just as you need to think clearly before making critical decisions in life. You consider your abilities, the course conditions, and your lie, or the position in which your ball comes to rest, with respect to your next shot, just as you would consider your talents and capabilities with respect to the challenges before you and how to make your next move in life. Perhaps you consider the hazards and the worst-case scenario as well as opportunities and your best possible miss should you not make the shot you intended. And good course management compels you to get your head into the game and to make an absolute decision with respect to your next play (or your next play in life). Gradually, this process reflects in your playing style and can result in incredible consistency and low scores. Your mind and body are working together.

In golf, you can break the overall winning strategy down into two main sections: mastering solid course management techniques and being able to visualize each shot. In the front nine, we will deal with various strategies for competitive play—the course management side of achieving your goals. When you use solid course management skills, you focus on making the right shot, the best one to make when considering your current skill level. You may know the course overall, but your focus is on dealing with one hazard at a time, and you consider each challenge individually. You approach it with the arsenal of fourteen weapons you carry in your golf bag—your putter, irons, and woods. Think of the clubs as the components crucial to your personal success action plan, the foundation of your positive working strategies, and the development of your winning habits.

The same holds true when you look at how to succeed in life. You step up and take the challenge, confident in your course management skills. You know what is required, you know what to do, and if you have been working hard to hone your skills, you know how to do it. The course management part of the success action plan encompasses knowing how to effectively use all the components detailed in the next nine holes to achieve your goals.

Your target? To turn aspirations into expectations.
Ready?

Swing Thoughts:

(A swing thought is a short catch phrase intended to help the player keep his or her mind in the game and focused on making the shot.)

Set goals and objectives
for self-improvement.

Develop a solid action plan and
be accountable and unbiased.

Evaluate and modify your plan
regularly and stay the course.

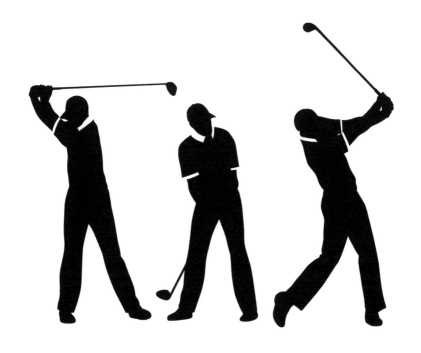

Course Management

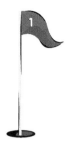

The 1ˢᵗ Hole – **Be Limitless**

People are complex and diverse beings, and our minds are amazing and powerful tools that need to be "worked." Although the brain is not a muscle, we need to train it as though it is. Think of building and flexing the brain like a muscle in order to elevate your level of knowledge, awareness, and brilliance. As is often said of muscle mass: use it or lose it! The brain is no different.

Today there is a wealth of research supporting the idea that you can take steps to stimulate and protect your mind. The key is continual learning. It starts when you are very young, snuggled in bed, listening to and imagining a story read by a parent or sibling, but continues well into your senior years when challenging your gray matter on a regular basis can actually mitigate the impact of aging and its effect on your thought processes.

Successful continual learning means maintaining a balance and variety of success-oriented attributes, the most prominent being awareness, confidence, persistence, determination, courage, and focus. But curiosity, ingenuity, and creativity may be even more important as it is these traits that fuel the desire to continue to question and challenge the status quo. In the chapters to follow we will explore how to embrace these valuable traits and incorporate them into day-to-day life. We will think and question and build as we go.

The secret to becoming limitless, where you are open to change and fresh ideas, involves finding that magical combination of inquisitiveness and determination that works for you personally. You then decide to work hard in order to achieve your goals in life while blocking obstacles that will slow your pace.

If I were to ask you to quickly jot down the traits that you value most in a successful person, you could probably rattle off at least ten without much effort. Some of those are likely the traits that got you to where you are today. But now what? What else do you want to do? *Where do you go from here?*

Barbell, book, or both

When you aspire to become limitless, both mentally and physically, it's never too late or too soon to pick up a barbell, book, or both.

———

The *barbell* represents any sort of physical activity. You need to make a conscious effort to include physical fitness in your life on a regular basis to prevent illnesses such as cancer, stroke, heart disease, and diabetes. A huge part of being physically healthy means avoiding a diet high in saturated fat.

Maintaining a good memory is directly linked to maintaining a healthy body. The *book* represents any form of mental activity—anything that challenges you, and preferably something you enjoy. Tackle a crossword puzzle, play a game of Scrabble, learn a new language, learn to play a musical instrument, or read a book. Get that brain stimulated and working. Increasing intellectual activity through formal and informal education and the resulting enhanced awareness can help you focus on your goals and steer clear of distraction.

The power behind the process

In order to achieve any high-level goals, it is crucial to establish a meaningful sense of self-worth and self-confidence, acknowledge known talents, and develop psychological skills. This is where the mind-body-achievement connection comes into play. The mind-body-achievement connection is the keen ability to be motivated and to push both your mind and body into high-functioning achievement mode.

So how does one sharpen this ability?

In any quest, there are two key motivators to be aware of that will play an important part in whether you are successful. First is your level of inherent interest, the extent to which you want to learn or know more about something or someone with respect to your goal. Second is your desire, the intensity with which you wish for or want something, or a specific outcome, again as related to your goal.

If your quest does hold a high level of interest and desire for you, the resolution to move forward and take action will naturally follow. At this point, being focused and strong mentally and physically, you can force your goals to take absolute priority. This is a learned process and one that can be perfected over time.

So let's delve into the development of the mind-body-achievement connection, using a big-picture approach. The power behind the mind-body-achievement connection process lies in the following three defining tasks. These will empower you and enable you to develop and work through the success action plan (SAP) for any target you may choose.

   o Replace unhealthful, detrimental behaviors with winning habits. This involves being

---

aware and willing to change, recognizing and depowering the impact of common excuses, and then ultimately eliminating them by upgrading to more favorable behavior.

o Develop a sense of self-worth, self-confidence, and lasting resilience. During the process of upgrading to winning habits, your sense of self will automatically evolve and upgrade.

o Build the psychological skills and mental toughness of a contender. Simple lifestyle changes over time will help you flex and build your self-control and willpower muscles and get your mind and body and achievement needs in sync. We will focus on exercising restraint and building discipline.

I choose to believe that the time is always right to learn something new, as long as you jump in at a level you're comfortable with. If you want to do something you know very little about, or if you have a wealth of knowledge about what you want to do, it's never too late or too soon. It's just the beginning.

You have no doubt heard the phrase "the light at the end of the tunnel." Like most clichés, it has a lot of truth in it. It can mean you are trudging along and then gradually everything becomes clearer, perhaps even wondrous by the end. But let's think about this. What if the light is at the beginning of the tunnel, and maybe it's not really a tunnel as we normally think of it—dark and cool and desolate. Maybe it's more of a channel that we work our way through, well lit throughout and acting as a positive, invaluable guide. You can never fall too far off course because there is a constant welcome reminder gently nudging you back in place so you stay on track and explore the limitless opportunities and possibilities before you.

The way I work at this is to begin with a full visualization of myself standing on the first tee box, looking down the fairway on my favorite golf course. The sun is brilliant, the weather perfect. I can smell the freshly manicured grass. I feel great. I am at the beginning of my game. I am limitless! My mind and body are ready to function in sync and I am focused on one achievement and goal—the win!

Now, join barbell and book together and see what happens: mental health and acuity begins to improve. New research strongly suggests mental and physical exercise of this nature may assist in the protection against or even prevention of mental decline such as Alzheimer's disease. It's hard not to want to jump in with both feet and believe; the merits of becoming healthier, mentally and physically, far outweigh any perceived risks.

Body, mind, spirit
Being at one with your world

Keeping in mind that maintaining a healthy brain is essential, and that entails giving it regular workouts, let's jump to the concept of becoming limitless and what it means to us in our everyday lives.

Becoming limitless involves training to be mentally and physically poised, with your mind and body working in harmony to achieve a targeted, successful outcome. It means going after and getting what you want.

Using the brain–muscle analogy, it can be seen that doing physical exercise and eating right promote mental and physical health and help the brain function more efficiently. As the brain and body act in unison, it stands to reason they should train in unison. It is about reciprocity—a healthy mind fuels a healthy body and a healthy body fuels a healthy mind, making your overall state of health the best it can be.

The human mind and body
are truly extraordinary.
They are the quintessence of
excellence in motion.
We talk, touch, see, hear, taste, smell, and feel.
We dream, aspire, and become.

All that we are is mind and body and spirit—that is our universe.

I don't want limits placed on my life or how I choose to live it, and I most certainly don't want self-inflicted limits. Thus the term *be limitless* holds great meaning for me. It means living a no-holds-barred, authentic life, in the moment and to the fullest.

As you stand at the tee box looking down the fairway toward your intended target, consider the following. There are hazards built into the course to restrict and challenge you. You can see them; they are intentional and legitimate. They are on the course guide and you will see them again and again as you play through each hole in the round. Yet even with all this information at your fingertips, they are still hazards. You are aware of them, but that doesn't mean you will always be able to avoid them. You have to work to reduce your exposure, and you have to strategize and practice to improve your game. You have to focus on building your abilities so you overcome the hazards.

Dealing with tangible, in-your-face hazards is a challenge in itself, but you must also think about the less tangible, unpredictable hazards, the ones that can get in the way and stop you short. This is the focus on the front nine: being able to recognize and face both tangible and unforeseen hazards—and excuses—in your daily life with ease.

Becoming limitless involves mental agility; the ability to quickly grasp and incorporate new ideas and concepts with confidence.

One of my favorite things about becoming limitless is the attraction to firsts and one-of-a-kinds. I am notorious for trying things that I have never done before. What is more exciting and invigorating than doing something for the first time? Of course, when we are young, this is an everyday occurrence. Yet as we grow and mature, the firsts happen less frequently as we gain more experience and expand our knowledge and perhaps become a little complacent. We often lose the drive to learn.

But if you are going to become limitless, you must summon the explorer within you. Try new things! Start at the beginning and push to learn about things of interest to you that perhaps you have been making excuses for not doing. Try something new—indulge! There is nothing like a new experience to stimulate the senses.

I thrive on creativity and challenge. As much as some things we do can develop into winning habits, sometimes it is not the act so much as the process that is the most important factor. The process of being limitless needs to become a habit. You are curious—to learn and create. So you feed your inquisitiveness and creativity, making it a priority in your life, committing to make time to explore, experience, and evolve. At this point, there is no room for self-induced limits.

One-of-a-kind situations, by definition, can happen only once, but often they are a modification of a first, where the activity continues but the process changes. For example, one summer I held cardboard boat races at our cottage. It was a get-together in which participants needed to be creative and innovative, building semi-functional boats out of cardboard, duct tape, and waterproof paint. It was incredible to see all the surprising designs that people came up with. Some boats were very stable and buoyant, and a real race took place as contestants rounded the last marker heading back to shore. Others were all about the appearance—pirate ships, a twenty-foot kayak complete with pontoon-like side floats and a banana boat so heavy it had to be brought in on a commercial trailer. Mix a little brilliance, elbow grease, and ingenuity together, add some healthy competition, and all of a sudden you have transformed refuse into floating works of art.

More recently, I held a similar event, a superhero party based on the 8th Hole chapter, "Become Unstoppable," from *Make it Happen*, the second book in the *3 Off the Tee* series. The activity was another get-together with friends, but the process changed from designing and building a semi-functional cardboard boat to creating original superheroes complete with costume, slogan, and special powers. Some people even had theme songs. It was a night filled with hilarity, and it was gratifying to see so much creativity.

Challenging people to be creative in a manner outside of their realm of expertise or even their comfort zone can often be exhilarating. This may be why I love the one-of-a-kind events. Fresh thinking needs to be embraced, and people get to do something new and be creative and perhaps try things that are out of character for them. There are just so many wonderful things to do in life, and that means sometimes we can only try things once before moving on to something else that's new. When we decide that we don't want to be stuck in repeat mode, we are ready to push beyond our limits.

How can you possibly do everything you want to do in life if you start doing a bunch of things twice?

If you start to do the same things over and over just for the sake of doing them as opposed to doing something to improve, you may be limiting yourself from exploring new experiences. And if you aren't enjoying yourself fully, you may be wasting time!

Of course, the point isn't necessarily to only have a cardboard boat race or a theme party once; it is to look at your daily life and start to analyze and then modify the habitual aspects.

The strategy of becoming limitless may begin with a first or a one-of-a-kind, but it is the thought process behind the event that is important. Gradually, you can get into the habit of doing something different each time you want a fun and varied experience. Not only will this help maintain a high level of interest, but it will also promote continual learning and curiosity.

Think about splitting your habits into two categories. If you are improving and learning, they are winning habits. If you are doing something just for the sake of doing it, they are time wasters. What activities do you fill your week with solely out of habit? How much time do you spend with your brain on autopilot, pursuing mediocre, time-filler types of activities? What do you wish you were doing with that time? Perhaps something awe-inspiring comes to mind—something limitless!

We all have familiar personal patterns—how we react, how we respond, and how we deal with life's difficulties. These patterns are generally comfortable and familiar and therefore we accept them. "This is who I am," we say, or "This is what I do."

However, this does not mean that these patterns are necessarily working in our favor. We could be holding ourselves back or falling into complacency by letting such familiar personal patterns continue without taking a closer look.

From time to time, it's important to shake things up a little. This facilitates the process of becoming limitless. You need to revisit habits that are not improving your life, break the pattern of making excuses, and trade up by replacing excuses with winning habits.

To drive or not to drive

I remember playing golf in Florida one year, where I was teamed up with a charming elderly lady. Then in her mid-eighties, she said, "It's a good day when my score beats my age!" And that day was a good day indeed as she shot eighty-one.

She went on to tell me that her father had been a great golfer, and she and her dad and her two brothers had golfed together from the time she could walk until she left home for university. "Those were the days!" she reminisced, "I was young and strong and limber. Today these old bones are brittle!"

She could no longer make the long shots nor twist her torso to swing through. She had altered her swing to mostly use her arms. She had retired her driver and now was hitting a shorter club off the tee. But she was consistent and accurate, and most importantly, she had adapted her game so she could play her best. At the end of the round she gave me a huge hug and the following advice: "Just remember to make every shot count!"

You become limitless when you overcome what holds you back.

Extend beyond your preconceived limits!

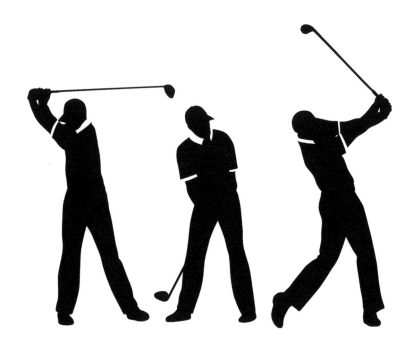

Course Management

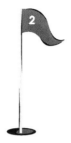

The 2ⁿᵈ Hole – **The Aerial Perspective**

Most golf scorecards include an aerial hole-by-hole view of their course as a course management guide for players. The map is an easily understood visual aid, a graphical overview that shows the course, its challenges, and complications. Offering a different perspective, the aerial view is of particular importance on holes that dog-leg left or right so you can't actually see your target, or where a multitude of hazards are at play.

The challenge for you in this chapter is to take an aerial perspective, a broader, more constructive, and unbiased overview, and apply it to personal achievement. To be constructive and unbiased when dealing with your own personal dreams and desires is not an easy task. Throw a little passion into the mix and you may be bursting with zealous enthusiasm, if you are achievement motivated, meaning you hold a strong, unflagging desire to succeed in life. Individuals of this nature usually want to achieve tasks of great importance, and when they do, they feel gratified. Laborious effort and extensive timelines are not considered daunting—the greater the challenge, the better it seems.

The flip side of being achievement motivated is being focused on failure avoidance. In these cases, the individual is more concerned with self-preservation and saving face. In order to avoid feeling incompetent or embarrassed, they steer away from challenge or give up too quickly, or they procrastinate and fail to give their best effort.

Because these are the extremes, you will likely agree that you fall somewhere in the middle, but you can alter how you think and gear up to create a motivational shift toward becoming more achievement motivated. Take on smaller challenges, build your confidence, and keep moving toward your targeted quest.

It starts with the aerial perspective. Stay focused on the constructive, unbiased overview of your goal. Stick to the facts and strip out emotion as you think. If you start to question and doubt anything about yourself or your goal, stop. Refocus specifically on the high-level goal only—its value and its merit.

Here are the keys to cultivating the beliefs required to achieve your goals:

- o Your success is your responsibility. Take the initiative, do the work, and persist to the end.

- o Think in terms of opportunities and solutions instead of problems, disappointment, and failure.

- o Value the effort you put forward. Be determined, committed, and involved.

- o Keep an open mind and know that you can always learn more.

- o Believe that your hard work, dedication and persistence will pay off; improve through continual learning and believe in your future.

If you are afraid to fail, your successes will be few, common, and unmemorable

Begin by looking at the big picture, the at-a-glance summary of what your target may look like, but do it with a *limitless* mindset. Focus on what you desire in life, whether personally or professionally, and ignore that little voice in your head chirping out objections. Here are some examples of goals many people seek:

o   Self-confidence and personal growth

o   Relationship and team building

o   Master planning and mentorship

o   Financial planning and wealth management

o   Professional directives and development

o   Effective business strategies

o   Fit lifestyle prototyping: a personalized pro-gram that focuses on strategically infusing a succession of small, incremental positive changes in your life that in time will become automatic winning habits and add up to big results that include improved quality of life, more energy, good health, and longev-ity. The success action plan for this goal will be detailed in Chapters 10 through 18.

I realize these are somewhat vague and all-encompassing points, but that is the intention. The idea for the model starts with brevity and then evolves and develops as you progress.

Again, if we look at the scorecard in golf, we recognize that the eighteen holes or segments are all challenging individually, and they are all integral to your overall success. You can't skip a hole because you parred it the last time, and you can't quit in midstream and return later. You commit to the challenge and you go for it, from beginning to finish. The game is yours, so you play to win.

Reinforcing the concept of beginning to end, alpha to omega, if you effectively negotiate your starting point, all the planned steps in the SAP are relevant and should not be skipped or discounted. Fast-track with vengeance, but steer clear of the shortcuts. Don't make excuses for why you're not doing what you have already deemed critical to your success.

Love thy competitor!

One of the interesting things about taking an aerial perspective is being able to look at things from a new angle, taking a fresh-set-of-eyes approach.

For instance, I have always worked in extremely competitive marketplaces where you watch your competitors and you watch your back. It's what I know.

Yet when I made the move to writing a few years back, I found I had to completely rethink the entire concept of the competitor. You see, a fellow author, writing in the same genre as you, is usually more of an ally than competitor. There is a sense of camaraderie and a well-accepted belief that you are stronger together. I might say, "Hey, if you like my book, you'll probably like this one too" when referring to another author's book. While friendly, positive competition is always a good thing, it doesn't have to mean your competitor is your enemy.

The aerial perspective allows this luxury. You can take a fresh look at your competition, unbiased and nonjudgmental.

Aerial Ops

From a distance, everything looks achievable, which is why it's so important to take the aerial perspective. The simple assumption is, "If this is what I want to do, I should just do it!" And you can, if you make realistic goal choices and you block excuses from limiting your potential.

From where you are now, looking forward, what do you see for your future—say, in one month, one year, or perhaps five years? Can you visualize what the future holds for you? Perhaps in one month you plan to have lost ten pounds, in one year you plan to have saved enough money for a deposit on your next house, or in five years you plan to be financially ready to start a family, to go back to school and earn your degree, or perhaps to send your children to college or university.

Sometimes it takes big dreams

Coming up with your aerial perspective is as simple as a one-line statement detailing what you want to achieve and then attaching a realistic timeline to it. You know there will be a beginning and an end with steps and challenges in between, but from a broad aerial perspective, the focus is more on what has to happen. It is the vision that includes details of how exactly the change will happen devoid of excuses, procrastination, and potential failure. It is all the irrepressible enthusiasm and gumption and resourcefulness you can muster rolled into a glorious ball of excitement. It starts with a clear sense of what your personal beginning is, what skills need to be developed, and a realistic sense of the time, cost, and commitment required.

I recently read an *Inc. Magazine* interview with Steve Jobs from 1989 where he was named Entrepreneur of the Decade. *Inc.* editors George Gendron and Bo Burlingham asked Jobs the following question:

INC.: You mean the technology is changing too fast?

Jobs: Yeah, and customers can't anticipate what the technology can do. They won't ask for things that they think are impossible. But the technology may be ahead of them. If you happen to mention something, they'll say, "Of course, I'll take that. Do you mean I can have that, too?" It sounds logical to ask customers what they want and then give it to them. But they rarely wind up getting what they really want that way.

It occurred to me that to think customers won't ask for things they believe are impossible may be a premise lost in today's world largely because of Job's contribution to technology. Aside from revolutionizing an industry, he and Apple have enabled us to question the relativity of the *impossible*. I recently listened as my eighty-eight-year-old father explained to my eldest brother that his new iPad was fast, had 64 GBs, and if he ran out of space he could store the data overflow on cloud. His concern? He had a lot of pictures and videos he wanted to use on his blog, and he didn't want to run out of space.

My father likes the iPad's ease of portability and being able to FaceTime friends and family, but most significantly, he looks forward to what will come next, how innovation and technology will again impact his life. He is thriving in the present and gleefully anticipating all that's *possible* in the near future.

I will achieve this on this timeline!

The limitless mind lets us dream and examine and explore. It opens us up to opportunity. We come up with a desire, a clear, fresh perspective, and a potential goal to observe from afar. And we wonder, is this it, the right choice, the best choice to follow?

Everything we do today has meaning, not only for this day but for all the days to follow. The way we spend each and every day has a definite impact on our future. Each day our focus and effort can bring us closer to what we desire.

Live in the present, but live for the future

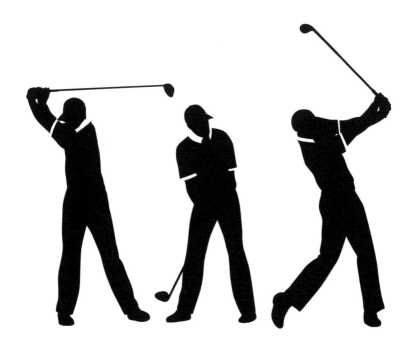

Course Management

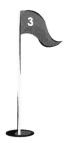

The 3rd Hole – **Aspirations**

What is your passion? Do you have a life purpose, or do you dream about doing something that would fulfill your life? I am certain that there is something very important to you, something that you have always wanted to do, a hope or ambition of achieving something in your life.

Have you already blurted out the answer, or is it trapped somewhere in the past, weighted down by overwhelming voices that drone, "I have to do this first" or "I just don't have the time or the talent"?

Aspire, ascend, soar, and excel!

The promise of aspiration is that it is evolutionary. The human condition is such that we are always aspiring to be something more, something better, something nobler. It starts as a thought, a want, a need, or a desire and then grows and evolves with intention and direction, upward with lust and hunger. The continued drive feeds the rise.

If your aerial perspective is to tackle the SAP by focusing on a lifestyle prototype of energy, health, and longevity, the next steps are to recognize and own your aspirations and then consider how you could tie those aspirations to direct, measurable, and documented expectations.

Here are some critical strategies to keep in mind:

o People aspire, learn, and grow when they are ready to commit to the process.

o People rise to the occasion without hesitation when they feel inspired and challenged.

o When aspirations are perceived to be achievable, ambition and drive can erase excuses.

o Core passions and aspirations should be consistent and in sync.

Aspirations start the process, then you access your beginning point, decide what needs to take place, and launch your quest, expecting to complete it on a specified timeline.

———

Around-the-couch crusading

Often when we feel frenzied and frustrated, we engage in reward-seeking behavior because we think it is going to make us feel good. Suppose you have had a stressful day and want to relax for a while. You sit on the couch and watch your favorite show, which leads to the next show, and the next, and you know you should get up and do something, but you don't. You end up living your life vicariously through your favorite TV actors instead of actually living your own life, and the only crusading you attempt is that trip to the fridge. Yikes!

When stress brings the onset of cravings, and you end up eating chips and dip, wings and beer, maybe some ice-cream and chocolate sauce, after the bingeing stops, the tendency is to not feel good at all, but to feel disappointed in yourself. The evening is shot and you are uncomfortably full and bloated, and that never feels good.

If your aspirations tend to run sideways from time to time, leaving you with no time or energy to pursue your dreams, you can actively work to exercise your willpower. We are not born with willpower; we learn it, build it, and master it.

If you come home stressed, by all means relax and watch your favorite show, but when it's over, force yourself to get up and do something.

———

The next time you are tempted to sabotage your aspirations, stop! Ask yourself how you are feeling—anxious, nervous, discouraged? How do you expect you will feel if you give in to temptation? Disappointed?

If you can indulge a little and feel good afterward, you are exercising some valid restraint. But if you overindulge and feel rotten afterward, then your perceived reward is really a punishment of sorts. You didn't feel so good in the first place, so you tried to make yourself feel better, but the approach you took did not work—so now what? Will you give up?

I often hear people complaining of their uncontrollable lack of willpower and overindulgences. When they are referring to wasting time and overeating, I ask, "How hungry are you?" Interestingly, after a puzzled look, the answer is almost always, "Oh, I'm not that hungry!" to which I ask, "Then why were you bingeing?"

If you want long-term results, you need to examine what is going on in your life that is causing you to tolerate *unrewarding*, destructive behavior. People are usually not stressed or hungry if they have a low activity level. Healthy people are generally not that unmotivated, despondent, and unhopeful unless they are not mindfully exercising their willpower to achieve things in their lives and feel better.

Here is a quick TV-time willpower-building trick. Sit on an exercise ball and balance with your feet up off the ground for as long as you can. Or, every time a commercial comes on, don't go to the fridge or pantry; instead, stand tall and alternate legs, lifting your knees up to your chest, and keeping your balance. You will become more active, less likely to binge, and you will actually end up relaxing and rewarding yourself, which was the original goal. These are simple, easy steps to exercise and flex your willpower.

Aspirations and inspiration go hand in hand

Now consider these questions:

o What do you want to achieve—today, this week, this year, in your lifetime?

o Are your aspirations tied to your core passion?

o Have you decided to foster and cultivate your aspirations and make them a priority for you?

o Do you truly believe that you can achieve them?

The gap between the initial aspiration and the expected outcome needs to be defined, aligned and challenged. Ask yourself why you feel the quest you have chosen is important to you and what you expect to happen. Think about what you have to gain in the near and distant future if you achieve your goals. You must be convinced that the quest is of definite value to you, so the first step is to convert your aspirations to expectations.

Filling the gap between aspirations and expectations is directly tied to the mind-body-achievement connection. We mentally and physically work our way through the process of aspiration, action, and ultimately achievement.

How can you improve your handicap if you don't know what it is?

In golf, a handicap is the average difference between at least ten rounds of a player's scores and a set standard for the course. For example, if your average score is 89 and par for the course is 72, then your handicap would be 17. It's like a benchmark; it's the best way to see whether you are improving. You know your handicap so you continually strive to play better. And when you play better, your average score is lowered; thus, your handicap is lowered.

You can reduce your handicap significantly if you have a consistent approach. If you work on improving all year long, if you have weaknesses

---

or restrictions, work on them. If you live in a climate where you can't golf all year long, use indoor driving ranges or work out to build your strength and flexibility. Keep your game in play all year long—"off-season" is not an excuse to stop. The extraordinary side effect of this kind of commitment and hard work is a resurgence of a sense of fulfillment and self-confidence.

The handicap levels the playing field overall, which allows you to focus on how you'll improve. How will you fill the gap between aspiration and expectation?

When we watch pro golfers, we expect them to play well, to make the shots we know we can't, and to be entertaining. Their expectation, however, is very different. They expect to succeed!

Grab hold of your aspirations, dust them off, and set them on a pedestal. Examine them and embrace them. Give them renewed importance and value. Give them new life. What do you want to create?

If your aspirational tap has been turned off for years, you may need to coax that first drip and encourage the trickle before you can really get it flowing, but that's okay. Again, remember that there are always beginning points no matter where you are in life. Begin at your beginning—just begin! The process—and real change—will follow.

You must be grounded to take flight

Successes in life don't happen for one reason, but many, and are usually the result of a lot of dedication and hard work. Those efforts often go unseen to the average spectator but they happened all the same. For example, take a new band that seemingly comes out of nowhere and goes on to achieve great levels of success. Only later do you discover that the band has been in the industry for years, working hard in obscurity, and the song that became an "instant hit" is actually on the band's fifth album that had gone mostly unnoticed along with the previous four albums until just recently. Was the band any less talented before its big hit?

This is also very true in the golf world. It takes years and years of hard work, practice, and determination to become consistently good at the game.

The limitless aerial perspective opens up immense opportunities. Aspiration backed with desire and passion, along with some well-exercised willpower, will set you on an upward track. Empowered by your new understanding of what truly makes you feel better—achievement rather than overindulgence—you are set in motion. Aspire, ascend, soar, and excel.

An aspirational diet will have you dreaming of success; but it's the attachment of expectations and tangible goals that feeds the desire, persistence, and fortitude required to make the win.

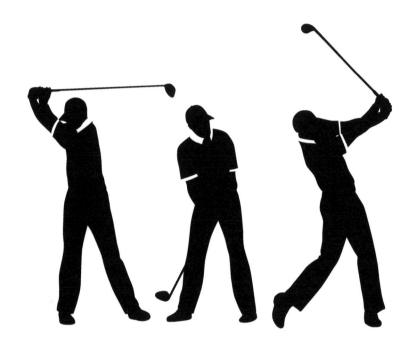

Course Management

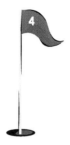

The 4th Hole – **Excuse Management**

I have been thinking about the idea of excuses for some time now. They are like menacing demons that creep into our lives without us knowing. They are roadblocks, white lies to ourselves, a reason to set the bar lower, and self-justification for achieving less than our full potential. An excuse is often a defensive effort to explain away a fault or an offense in the hope of being forgiven or understood.

But if you need to be forgiven for something, you should apologize, not make excuses. If you need to be understood, you should explain yourself, not make excuses. If you are making excuses, you need to ask yourself why.

When you actively take measures to manage what is controllable in your life, you'll find that you stop making excuses. Fully engaged and strategically focused on your intended target, you drive your ball toward the best possible outcome—and you forget about making excuses. It may not be your final destination, but at least you are in control and out of excuse-making mode.

The nature of the excuse

The threat to our well-being when we make everyday excuses is subtle, insidious, and ever-present. Defensiveness and excuse-making wear us down gradually and steal our zest for life. Excuse-making on a habitual basis has a powerful, negative effect on people who don't know they're doing it—a stalling effect that kills momentum.

To become mentally strong and fit, you need to stop making excuses and take responsibility for your actions. I call this "excuse management." Managing excuses means not excusing yourself from the responsibility you need to take with your thoughts, words, and actions.

The hardest part is becoming aware of and identifying when you're being defensive and making excuses. This requires you to be brutally honest with yourself. At first, you may not even recognize when you're doing it. Ask your family and friends to help out. Gradually, you'll start to be aware of the difference between valid reasons for doing something and making excuses or being defensive.

Self-obsess less

As I've indicated, the first thing to consider when dealing with excuses is that you need to be self-aware so you can identify them. Next, you need to arm yourself with winning habits so you can move beyond their limitations. And finally, you have to manage them so they don't creep back into your life again and again.

Applying these steps to your daily life has many positive side effects. One of the most interesting is that you'll find you have little to no time left to self-obsess and worry about what you can't or won't do and then have to make excuses for it later. What a load off!

Excellence over excuses

I wholeheartedly believe that if you focus on excellence, gradually you will fall out of the excuse habit. Start by considering and reflecting when you say things like, "Yeah, that sounds pretty exciting, but I could never do that!" or "Yes, she is amazing. I wish I'd had the same opportunities." If these refer to something that you really want to do yourself, they are excuses.

Here's another example. A good friend has said to me several times over the years, "I love the relationship you have with your husband.

45

You're like best friends. I want the same kind of relationship, but my wife and I fight all the time and we can't stop." Funny, his wife says the same thing to me, but they don't say it to each other and they don't make changes. They have just one excuse for their inability to improve their relationship, one they repeat and reinforce until it's entrenched in their thinking. "We argue and fight all the time and we can't stop!" It's as though they have resigned themselves to the fact that the situation is completely out of their control, using the same feeble excuse over and over until they truly believe there are no other options.

So, how do they change their situation? They have to begin by first recognizing their excuse and working to banish it. Next, they have to believe they can make positive changes, then take action on those beliefs.

Another example: if you want to advance in your career and take on a more assertive role, you'll need to work on revitalizing your self-image so you can feel confident in achieving your objective. Your sub-consciousness, where your inner confidence resides, and your consciousness need to be aligned and working in tandem. Again, being aware and taking small steps to gradually develop winning habits will lead to reflexive positive responses. As you see and feel that you are acting and responding in a more positive manner and not falling victim to ordinary, unwanted excuses, you will feel revitalized and in control.

Usually the biggest difficulty in moving beyond excuses occurs when we act in a manner that contradicts what we are feeling inside. If you have a low sense of self-worth or an inaccurate inner image, and your self-worth and inner image do not match what you want to create in your life, then moving beyond excuses will be difficult.

Excuse management prerequisites

It's one thing to make excuses for what you don't want to do; it's another thing altogether to make excuses for why you're not doing what you do want to do.

Many people make excuses every day—some to save face, some to avoid judgment or even ridicule, and some to avoid disappointing or hurting others. But the ones that are detrimental and destructive are the ones that are limiting your potential. Once you become aware of the excuses you harbor and their potential detriment, you will start to understand the need to stop making them.

If you break down your excuses, you may find they fall into three main categories: fear, laziness, and procrastination of the stuff you don't want to do right now. Of these, the worst culprit is fear. Fear can mean a fear of failure, fear of rejection, or fear of loss; any of these three can be so debilitating that you can end up trapped on the excuse hamster wheel if you aren't careful.

At this point, you are probably becoming more aware of the excuses you make, and you may have a few in mind that you have decided to target. Write them down and review the list often. Overcoming the habit of making excuses is just like breaking any other habit: it takes work and repetition. Replace your old excuse habit with new, more positive mental habits.

The ball doesn't judge me, so why should I judge myself?

Aerodynamic, symmetrical, and resilient, the golf ball can take whatever you've got to give it. It's a symbiotic and mutually respectful relationship: you take your best shot and whether you hit or miss, there will be no judgment.

Not feeling judged is invaluable in life too. Imagine being able to speak truthfully about anything that is important to you and not be judged! This feeling is freeing, invigorating, and truly empowering, but so often it is undermined by insecurity and low self-esteem and other factors. It is human nature to judge others, and it's often hard to avoid judgment in everyday life.

Sometimes we make excuses for what we have done, knowing in our hearts that we did it intentionally because we wanted to, but also knowing that telling others the truth might lead to being judged. We are judged in both casual and long-term, deeper relationships. We are judged every day.

Judging by the terror on your face, you must be afraid of something

Do you judge others because you genuinely care about them and respectfully want the best for them, or do you simply do it out of habit? Consider the fact that judging takes time—a lot of time. So why would you spend precious time judging others?

Do you judge yourself? Do you judge yourself too harshly and too often? Do you worry that others are judging you? If so, this time-wasting habit is restricting your ability to aspire to better things. Make the decision to move forward and take the power out of your fear of being judged.

I love the idea of not being judged by others and not judging myself. I push myself into what I call *auto-aspire* mode: raising my subconscious level so I am open to exploring the value of aspirations and it becomes automatic. I need to feel totally free and open to dream and fantasize and follow the scent of a quest, one that may be so subtle initially that I have yet to truly understand my desire to pursue it and what opportunities may come forth. This is why I like the idea of playing a round of golf with my nonjudgmental golf ball. It's a welcome break. Don't use the fear of being judged as an excuse that holds you back.

Excuse Management 101

Let's discuss the tools we need to manage excuses. They include visualization and focus. The process is straightforward; there's no big secret or mystery. You just need to manage your excuses and take control.

STEP 1: Identify. Make a list of all the excuses you can think of that creep into your life in the course of a day. How many excuses are you tolerating?

o No time

o No money

o No experience

o No knowledge

o No talent

o No real desire

STEP 2: Analyze. Review your excuses and divide them into categories based on the following questions. Are they valid? Are they realistic? Are they self-inflicted? Are they limiting your success potential?

STEP 3: Manage. Make a concentrated effort to deal with the excuses you regard as detrimental to your ongoing success track.

STEP 4: Mitigate. Banish the outdated excuses that are stifling your authentic productivity.

There is only room in your life for positive energy. Focus on becoming limitless. This is *your* success action plan!

Excuses fall silent behind self-control, focus, and direction.
Once your excuses are gone, you will simply have to settle for being awesome!

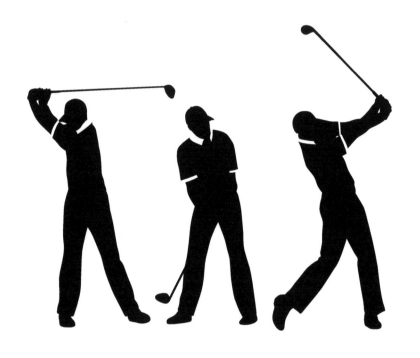

Course Management

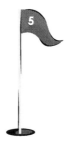

The 5th Hole – **The BIG Push**

As a kid, I would rush home from public school and my Mom would ask, "What new thing did you learn today?" As soon as I learned this new game, I was eager to play. So I would pay a little more attention at school and come home armed with answers that I was certain would impress. I wanted to be smart! I wanted to be interesting! Thank you, Mom, for instilling a lifelong love of learning in me.

As a young adult, I added a question myself: "What new thing did you do today?" My intention was to scrounge up some sort of new activity, something physical or creative, something different from the day or days before.

If I challenge myself in this manner every day, I am proactively pushing myself to be not only limitless and aspirational but acutely aware of how I am spending my time and how I am honing my ability to achieve.

Brainstorm Interpret Go (BIG)

So what is the BIG push? BIG stands for Brainstorm, Interpret, Go. It means being proactive. It is the decision to initiate positive change on a continuing basis. The best way to illustrate this is to look at any pro athlete. They practice and push in order to achieve. They don't give up. They brainstorm, considering what it will take for them to have the edge or advantage, then they interpret how they can perfect both their mental and physical strategies and put into practice their personal playbook of endurance drills. And then, most importantly, they act, proactively doing the work and gravitating toward the win.

An example of positive, self-induced, proactive change would be getting in shape because you want to, not because your lack of ambition got the best of you. You keep the odds of success in your favor by invoking positive change.

The BIG push means being able to develop and sustain momentum toward your goal; it is the process of actively replacing excuses with winning habits, the ultimate excuse blockers. Moreover, it is being willing to go to the wall for what you want or believe in, to push beyond your previous mental and physical limits, no matter what it takes.

Early in the process, and just when you think you are starting to make progress, you may become tempted to take a break or a time out. Sometimes this is what's needed, but other times, when you are building winning habits, certain guidelines should be adhered to.

You need a minimum committment of sixty hours, equally spread over a ten week period to push your positive routines and activities to the winning-habit level. You begin, you press on, and you endure without letting anything impede your progress, all the while advancing toward your goals. The BIG push actually kicks in after you have winning habits in place—it is the desire to take yourself to the next level.

What is your BIG push for today, this week, this month, this year?

Push today for what you want tomorrow!

I have a relentless sense of confidence. I believe I can do anything I put my mind to. If I want to do something, I think about it, visualize it, research it, and internalize the process until a game plan detailing the gap between where I am now and where I want to be crystallizes into an action plan. I see the challenge and immediately push to come up with my best plan to get there. I push and I push hard. My desires take priority.

In golf, if you want to break 100, 90, 80, or 70, you need to be consistent. You need to be able to repeatedly make the same shot on demand to lower your score.

The five fundamentals that lead to consistency are your grip, your ball position, your alignment, your tension level, and your balance from address to the end of your follow-through. The best place to strengthen your abilities and develop your proficiency is at the driving range. Many people have their favorite practice and warm-up drills in golf and swear by them.

Equally important are the practice and warm-up drills in life. It is these types of daily drills that keep us determined over the long haul, forging ahead on purpose with purpose. Practice and drills help prevent excuses from piling up, which only deplete willpower and allow susceptibility to failure.

Honing endurance and push drills

A great golf example of honing an endurance drill is putting practice. I putt repeatedly from various distances and slopes on a practice green to warm up and get the feel and speed down. I alternate with a push drill that starts ten to fifteen yards from the hole. I may take fifty shots at this distance before moving one meter closer and continuing with another fifty shots. As I move closer to the hole, the shots are much easier.

The long putts are how I push myself in this case. I could have started closer and worked my way farther from the hole, but I find that starting at the most difficult position allows me to improve my accuracy more quickly. I don't harshly judge my performance as I know I am starting at a more difficult level, and I don't make excuses because I know I haven't yet warmed up. I own 100 percent of my focus.

What did you learn today?
What did you do today that was different from the day or days before?

Here's another example. I often tackle learning new languages when I travel abroad. My preferred method is to use Rosetta Stone software in the correct dialect for my destination. I set my preferences and begin. I could simply work through the lessons one by one and work on my accuracy; instead, I push ahead in order to fast-track my progress and blast past my previous limits. I start at lesson one and continue for a time period of an hour or even longer if I have the time, and I remain alert. Rather than stopping and going back to lesson one and repeating it until I fully comprehend every last detail, I forge on.

Now, you would think my comprehension level would decline so rapidly that this would be a waste of time. But due to the way the software repeats and builds on concepts, quite often the content introduced in the first lesson is reinforced in lesson two and so on, and often subtle differentiation becomes more apparent moving forward.

Once my time allotment or concentration level has run out, I pack it in for the day. The next day, I begin at the first lesson again and continue in the same manner. Lesson one will stay in my routine until I feel I have mastered it. Then it will drop off. I will continue to add new material, dropping off the oldest, already learned material as I push to complete the entire program.

Each day I push further as I know more, and the process becomes easier for me. Once again, though, I don't harshly judge my language skills as I am tackling a language new to me, and I don't make excuses because I know I am pushing myself hard and seeing rapid advancement. I am focused on learning, not being perfect, especially at this level. The most important point, again, is that I own 100 percent of my focus.

In both of these examples, the endurance drills require the use of psychological skills to encourage performance improvement.

———

***This is about me being ready to succeed.
When I win in my mind, I truly win.
Anything worthwhile deserves some time.
I will do it this time! No excuses!***

The BIG push comes after embracing your aspirations, working to fill any knowledge or skills gaps, and tying your expectations to your aspirations. It is the process of pushing beyond known limits, whether mental or physical.

If you've been following me, at this point you know what you want and you believe you can achieve it. You are also aware of excuses that may come into play, and you banish them and commit to forging ahead, using positive winning-habit routines and activities. You push yourself every day to develop your endurance drills, and ultimately, you're able to concentrate your effort on a particular goal.

If you know what you're up against, you can plan. If you can plan, you can win. This is true on the golf course, where you use good course management practices, and it's true for every other aspect of life. In golf, your ultimate goal is to lower your score—a low score means success. To get there, you use your practice plan or strategy in order to define how you are going to achieve your goal. You need to know what clubs to hit, how far you hit the ball with them, and be proficient at working the ball to your advantage. There is so much that you can do—when you have a plan.

If you take a moment to think of someone who has really impressed you, you will no doubt have a sense of what the BIG push looks like. It is a process not to be taken lightly. I find that the people I know who have this powerful sense of dedication, force, and conviction have worked to take their willpower and confidence to a new level. They have proactively pushed themselves to be their best, time and time again.

Go BIG or go BIG . . . there is nothing else!

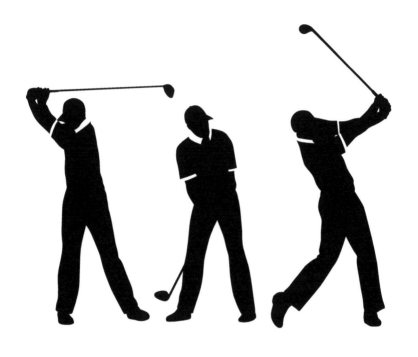

Course Management

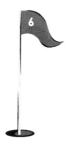

The 6th Hole – **Motivation**

According to Wikipedia, "motivation is the psychological feature that arouses an organism to action toward a desired goal and elicits, controls, and sustains certain goal-directed behaviors. It can be considered a driving force; a psychological drive that compels or reinforces an action toward a desired goal." A successful motivation strategy deals with potential deviations while encouraging you to stay the course and get back on track as fast as possible if you stray. It is the driving force that gives you the will to continue, to forge ahead and fulfill your wants and needs. It is the fuel of your desires.

Change how you think and feel and act and react

For most people, going three off the tee is one of the worst situations they can find themselves in on the golf course. That being said, you may question why I would name my book series *3 Off the Tee*—but there is a good reason. When I first took up golf, because I certainly didn't want to go three off the tee, I realized that the threat became less daunting when I felt and thought about it in a fresh way.

Much of what we do in life is directly affected by how we think and feel and react. In this case, I chose to view going three off the tee not as a horrible failure but as a positive sense of urgency, a time to regroup and refocus. It was not the time to get frazzled or lose my perspective, my pacing, and possibly the game.

If you are open to finding a fresh perspective and altering how you think and feel about, and how you react to, what is going on around you, whether it is good or bad, you can positively alter how you act and react.

It is often said that the game of golf is 90 percent mental—the strategy of how you "think" your way around the course needs to be your predominant focus. It is the strength of your desire to achieve your goal that will set you apart from the competition.

The year leading up to the next big age plateau can frighten the best of us 20, 30, 40, 50, 60, 70...

We are changing every second, every minute, every hour, and this change is subtle when viewed from a long perspective. But upon approaching a birthday marking another full decade of life, most of us start to view change in a new light. We are no doubt concerned about aging, and perhaps we are disappointed that some critical change we had planned for and counted on has not been realized. Perhaps the change we desired is coming too slowly or not at all. Yet change is necessary to personal growth through new experiences and challenges. If we don't change, we may keep repeating the same mistakes, year after year. The pursuit of new experiences—accepting challenges, creating, exploring—is invaluable to becoming a better, happier human being.

Let your passion in life be as conspicuous as the devilish grin on your face

Have you ever wondered why some people are successful at almost everything they do? Where does their drive and energy come from? How do they persist and endure and push on even in the face of repeated failure to that ultimate goal, when most people would have given up?

Motivation is the force that initiates, guides, and sustains our achievement-oriented behavior over time. It is what causes us to decide to take action, be willing to commit, and stick with our goals even when we experience setbacks. The force behind motivation can be biological, social, emotional or cognitive in nature.

Most of us are in pursuit of some kind of goal, seeking excellence in one or more areas in our lives, and that is the basis of our motivation. We want to be successful. For this reason, motivation is an area of psychology that commands much attention. We are trying to capture and realize that special combination of direction and drive that will positively affect how we pursue and achieve our goals.

Over the years, researchers have developed different theories to explain motivation. Here are three major theories of motivation as they relate to understanding the basis of our mental and physical desires and how we can strive to increase our chances for success.

The acquired needs theory: The most common theory of motivation is the drive toward specific, tangible and external goals: achievement, affiliation, and power. Achievement refers to the desire to demonstrate our competence. Because we are all somewhat selfish by nature, we desire praise for a job well done. Affiliation is more community based in that we are motivated by those around us—our friends, colleagues, team—to work together to get results. And lastly, we strive for power, another selfish desire, and we complete tasks in order to achieve a feeling or sense of authority.

The control theory: The control theory refers to the internal drive to try to dominate specific segments of our surroundings that we feel we can control. We pursue certain tasks based on our ability to control the outcome. This is very different from being power driven. We don't want authority necessarily, we want order and predictability.

The expectancy theory: This motivation theory examines the nature of the goal. We as the goal seeker want to be perceived as competent, and thus we are drawn to goals that are safe and achievable. We have specific expectations: what's in it for me, will there be little frustration, and finally, will fulfilling the task showcase my competence?

The adage of self-motivation, the rules of consent

The power that drives us to push on diligently and persistently is self-motivation. Founded on the desire to continue learning and the need to succeed, it is a primary means of goal realization and individual growth. Self-motivation is closely related to our ability to be inventive and generate goals that sustain our interests and passions. We trust that we have the required skills and competencies to achieve our goals so we commit our efforts to doing so.

Self-motivation techniques:

Talk the talk. Share your goal and aspirations with those of like minds, perhaps someone optimistic and supportive whom you see as a mentor.

Keep a positive mind. Remember, a failed attempt doesn't make you a failure—giving up does.

Accentuate your interests. It is always easier if you are genuinely interested in achieving a set goal or task, yet you may sometimes find yourself in a position where you need to complete daunting tasks to allow you to move on to the next level of a larger goal. If this is the case, realign your focus to look forward to what is to come after the difficult step has been successfully completed.

Blueprint your success. What are you working on? What is the timeline? Is your goal realistic? How are you progressing? Are you ahead of schedule?

Energize to the skies. Get on the healthy track: proper sleep, exercise, balanced nutrition, and hydration will keep you sharp and up for the challenges.

Pay it forward. Assist, support, and encourage others to achieve their goals.

Encourage a lifestyle of learning.

Gain headway with challenge *chunking:* Smaller, easy to accomplish goals are tackled first. Then you progress to more difficult challenges and over time you build some kick-ass confidence. Think of the big picture in terms of a successful succession of smaller goals en route to eventually achieving a bigger goal.

I trust I will do what I put my mind and body to

The fear-of-failure concept can take on a new flavor if you consider the following. You can be successful and happy without being perfect. Making mistakes is normal; trying to correct them is what matters, the solution matters. Do your best in everything you do, even if it falls short of perfection, instead of struggling to excel at one thing.

Whatever you find to be limiting your progress is a form of excuse, which can hinder your motivation. Once you are aware of it, consider how you can think differently about it.

When you are open to change, your attitude changes, and you alter your behavior and rework your lifestyle. You are open-minded yet selective—what works remains, what doesn't gets revisited, and challenges get revised or discarded. But all the while you continue to push on.

———

Aspire to high standards, expect strong results, offer self praise, and stack your confidence

The motivation cycle begins with goal setting. You travel step by step toward your goal. You set daily, weekly, monthly, and annual goals that are measurable and flexible. You keep score and stay in the moment even while keeping your goals in mind. You establish new, consistent routines to support change and set a safety threshold so you can't falter too long or lose your way. And you regularly acknowledge effort and success.

It is important to note that it is *you* who must set your goals and then *you* who must achieve them. If I or anyone else were to set goals for you, you could come up with a gazillion excuses why they are not attainable. But that's not how it works. The motivation needs to come from within you.

The Weighted Stack

When you take each of your achievements, no matter what their independent value, and stack them one by one, you continue to build their overall impact. Viewed together, small changes and improvements add up.

In order to achieve peak performance, you need ongoing high motivation. The more daunting your quest, the more important your motivation becomes.

When you apply appropriate motivation to your aspirations and expectations, you improve the probability of success. It is that little nudge that says, "Hey, don't give up—you really want this!" There is weight—you want something and you know why. You are spreading out and reaching for what you truly value and want. You are self-motivated.

Over time, consistent motivation helps you to develop winning habits and use them to replace excuses. You go after what you want in life almost instinctively, and you gradually build your confidence.

Tell yourself often:
I am going to tackle my aspirations
head on with the passion
and dedication necessary to exceed
even my expectations

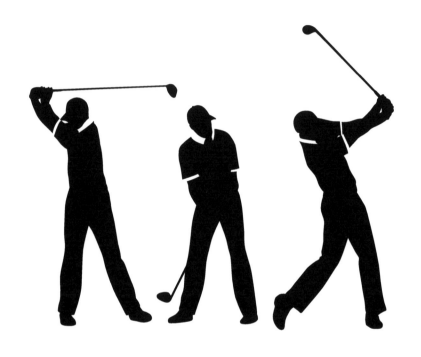

Course Management

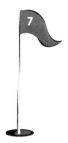

The 7th Hole – Inspiration and Incentive

In my early twenties, as an aspiring singer/songwriter, I took a recreational singing course. It was a popular class that attracted a diverse mix of people, all with very different expectations of what new skill they might take away.

I had signed up for the course for fun and a break from my heavy course load at the time, and I had no real expectations. But others had aspirations of grandeur of varying degrees. One girl was going to be performing on a televised singing competition, had the jitters, and couldn't hit the high notes in the song she had chosen. Four people were practicing for a company skit in which they had to act and sing in front of their colleagues. Three younger guys in a band were looking to gain some confidence and stage presence as performers, and an older gentleman with a nice speaking voice amused me when he sang with an annoying nasally twang.

Initially, I had thought this would be just a fun, light-hearted class, but it didn't take long for me to realize that there was a lot more going on. You see, the instructor turned out to be remarkable—knowledgeable and intuitive—and a great help to each member of the group. He was inspirational.

What's in it for me?

Each week, I observed as he worked with individuals in the class and helped them to make great leaps forward in their abilities. I saw him ask strategic questions, drilling down to out find why each of us was taking the course. Then he would delve, one person at a time, into what we expected to take away from the course, focusing on just two or three students per class. It was interesting how he would use this information to encourage and inspire us to overcome our fears, insecurities, and shortcomings to push us to be the entertainers that we all longed to be.

Week by week, as I watched him help others transform, I became increasingly confident that he would also help me, and so I looked forward to each class that much more, wanting the change for myself. The competent coach, who genuinely wanted to help others succeed, used his expertise to assist and inspire individuals in the class to reach their specific goals. The incentive or reward the coach provided was constructively building our confidence—in ourselves and in our abilities to perform and entertain.

The significance here is that all incentives begin with the recipient asking themselves one very pointed question: what's in it for me? If the answer is readily found, you may be inspired and motivated to continue.

Public speaking becomes easy when it's a topic you're genuinely passionate about

The instructor's words of wisdom went something like this: "If you can become comfortable singing in front of others, which you seldom do, you will undoubtedly become more comfortable speaking in front of others, even when you speak to people in everyday life."

Instead of a fun break, this singing class became a journey of self-discovery for me. I was intrigued and inspired by this man. He motivated and encouraged me to upgrade my skills in singing in front of a group and, by association, speaking in front of a group, skills not addressed in any of my regular curriculum. He inspired me to wonder, could I sing, could I write music, could I play guitar well enough? I wanted to find out!

The goal? I loved music and wanted to be good at performing. The inspiration? Here I was with access to a wonderful coach and in the company of others who had the same interests as I did. I was immersed in a magnificent, compassionate pool of learning and support. The incentive? Anticipation of the payoff: To be able to sing and play songs I had written. I was learning and improving, while honing my skills.

Incentives create motivation for behavioral change, both good...

Incentives work well when they are properly structured, monitored, and administered. They must be realistic, attainable, and of benefit either singularly or mutually to those involved. If an incentive plan is layered over an effective action-oriented strategy, it will reinforce the force and flow of the strategy. There needs to be opportunity, inspiration, motivation, incentive, and ultimately knowledge that the outcome is attainable.

Consider the following:

Opportunity: To enter a golf competition.

Inspiration: Annika Sorenstan, her abilities and legacy.

Motivation: I am determined to excel at a sport I love.

Incentive: To win a golf competition.

Desired Outcome: To improve my skill-sets, both mental and physical.

Here's another example:

Opportunity: To gain market share.

Inspiration: A close look at the competition.

Motivation: To build a successful business.

Incentive: Develop a bonus structure for all levels of staff.

Desired Outcome: Improved productivity and profitability overall.

And bad...

Ideally, the plan is to increase performance by increasing motivation. Sounds straightforward, right? But building an effective incentive plan usually involves substantial investment and quite often can backfire a few times before all the bugs are worked out. Several times over the years, I have seen well-intended business incentive plans that have gone very wrong.

There are various reasons to implement an effective incentive plan specifically designed to suit your targeted audience:

o To convert failure, or the potential for failure, into success

o To improve behavior and/or performance

o To engage and challenge employees

o To improve camaraderie and morale

o To retain talented and/or promising employees

o To increase individual, team, or management efficacy

Keep the focus by offering intermittent positive reinforcement en route to attaining larger goals

A well-orchestrated incentive plan addresses the following objectives:

o To change behavior

o To analyze and evaluate factors that affect that behavior, such as, skills, talents, motivation, and recognition. Then include them in a strategy to change behavior

o To develop a full and meaningful comprehension of the targeted goal(s) o   To detail process benchmarks to be used to measure progress

o   To clearly answer the question of "What's in it for me?"

o   To promote or encourage gradual, continual focus on attaining the original goal

Pay yourself forward for success

Our lives are full of incentives to motivate us. If you work smarter, you will get that promotion, and then you will be able to afford that trip, a new car, or a new house. These kinds of incentives are actually quite effective as long as you stay focused on rewarding yourself for your successes.

Let's say you are having car problems. Your personal incentive plan is that you are going to earn a promotion with better pay and then reward yourself with a new car, one that you have been admiring for some time.

At this point, there is no promotion on the horizon, but despite knowing that, you convince yourself that because you are having car problems— whether minor or significant—that you need that car *now*, and you can't wait for a promotion. Now see what you've done? You just turned your car problems into an excuse and overturned your personal incentive plan, rendering it of little or no value.

Rewards programs that work

My father worked for an innovative company that did two critical things right when inspiring its personnel. The first was the company's policy of having each new employee take a medical physical exam, and that same employee would have another physical upon retirement. The physical on the way in ensured that the employee was in reasonably good health, but the physical on the way out? If a health issue was found, the company would assist the employee in a way that left him or her with a clear plan to become more health conscious.

Granted, it would have been better for my father to have gone for physicals at regular intervals over the years, but he did not, and I suspect that few of his colleagues did either. Then one summer vacation, shortly before he decided to retire, four of his trusted friends and workmates had taken ill suddenly, all within their mid-forties to mid-sixties. The biggest culprit was heart disease. As a result, my father was more open to taking the physical and to the prospect of taking an early retirement.

His physical exam identified that he had high cholesterol and he was told he needed to exercise, dramatically alter his diet, and lose weight, which he did within the six months leading up to his retirement.

At my father's company, you could also earn points for your ideas and suggestions and use them to retire earlier with a full pension. All ideas and suggestions to increase productivity and/or profitability had to be written up on a proper form in detail, signed and dated, and submitted via suggestion boxes strategically located within the facility. Suggestions were taken seriously, and it was an honor to have yours considered. If a suggestion had value on its own merit or if there was potential for it to benefit the company, it was proposed for consideration. Ultimately, approved suggestions would involve collaboration, but credit was given where credit was due, including to my father. As a result, he retired early and healthy.

Create opportunities for success, then be inspired and motivated to go after them!

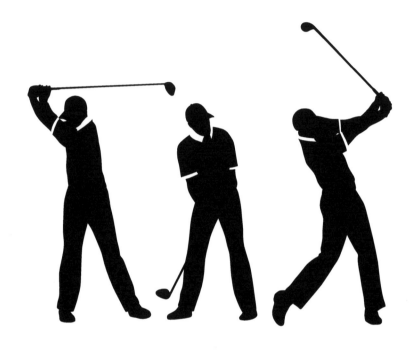

Course Management

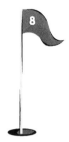

The 8ᵗʰ Hole – **The Vision**

In college, I studied psychology, religion, mythology, and philosophy in addition to business. I was trying to open my mind, to learn and absorb, to devour all things intellectual, and to develop my own interpretation. I read a book called *Man's Search for Meaning* by Viktor Emil Frankl: an Austrian neurologist, psychiatrist, and Holocaust survivor. Through his horrific experiences surviving two-and-a-half years in concentration camps, including Auschwitz, he struggled to find a reason to live and to find meaning in all forms of existence, even the worst imaginable. When he recognizes a human bone in the soup he and the other prisoners are being fed, I cannot even begin to imagine the horror and despair they must have endured.

Yet Dr. Frankl approaches his situation from a psychological perspective. He observes how the different prisoners (men in this case, because men and women were separated at the camps) react to their experiences, the effects of being dehumanized to the point of being known only as a number, their names long forgotten, the distress of not being in contact with loved ones or knowing of their safety, having to face the fact that they might be forced to live out the balance of their lives as slave laborers in the concentration camps, and knowing that any sign of weakness or illness would make for a very short life.

Dr. Frankl manages to mentally transport himself away from the stench of death and decay to a happier time and place so defined and vivid that he can absolutely smell the scent of fresh-cut grass around him and feel physically well and strong instead of malnourished and depleted. In this manner, he describes how finding meaning in life, or a reason to live, was imperative to surviving the camp.

From his experiences, Dr. Frankl developed the theory that man is driven by his search for meaning in life, and that the need for meaning seems to outweigh our unconscious desires.

From within the mind we look out and envision, contemplating and interpreting each new challenge and the action we will take

Aside from the moving account of Frankl's life in Auschwitz, which was so important on so many levels, his vision of normalcy and life became the beacon that has resounded with me since I first read his book—his desire for meaning, his reasons to live, and his vision of what it would be like on the other side, having survived such atrocities. Frankl's vision was tied to survival, but a fine-tuned vision in life can be tied to any goal you choose.

When we are fully engaged and moving toward our goals, it is because we have clearly identified the end point and the steps required to get there. A well-thought-out quest is best aided using goal-oriented visualization and mental-imaging techniques and using and working the mind-body-achievement connection, which is critical to success.

The mind and body working in tandem

When trying to improve in golf, you work through a series of drills to correct or enhance your abilities. You envision and then work toward achieving the goal you have set for yourself.

What keeps you sharp is the ability to acknowledge what the most difficult shot looks like whether on the course, at work, or in life. Think about this carefully. No matter how much planning, practicing, and analyzing you do, you will never be able to control all the variables. So you envision and practice what you want to happen, occasionally doing so from the perspective of getting out of the worst position you could possibly be in. Your vision needs to be ever-present in your mind and powerful enough to aid in cutting through the obstacles and roadblocks that could break your momentum.

Visualization is a creative effort. You imagine and cultivate every detail about something you want to achieve to create lasting mental pictures of yourself achieving your goals or improving your performance. When you imagine yourself achieving something, your brain will work to find a way to make it happen. It is like a mental rehearsal for success.

In whatever we do, we are influenced by past experiences. Family, education, travel, media, literature, and surroundings have all contributed to our life experience to date. Think of visualization as a portal to transport yourself to the place where you want to be. Think of it as being the polish on believing in yourself, your project or your goals. When you envision an outcome in such a way as it reinforces your belief, you reinforce your potential for success.

For instance, let's say you are terrified of speaking at an upcoming company meeting. Your belief, from past experience, is that you are not a good speaker. Perhaps in smaller groups you can muddle through, but in larger crowds you become so nervous and uncomfortable that the audience is also nervous and uncomfortable and hoping for the end.

If your vision is to move beyond the angst you feel and to believe that you are a brilliant speaker, you will have to set the stage in your mind. You'll need to create a new visual to support your more positive beliefs so your subconscious mind can get on board and you can improve.

Visualization is a very powerful tool, but only when your vision is in line with your beliefs. You will know when this is the case because you will entertain positive thoughts confirming your vision instead of negative ones that contradict your quest.

In the example above, two probable outcomes are 1) that you become a brilliant speaker or at least a good one, and 2) that you reduce you anxiety levels and feel better about yourself and your abilities.

The sweet spot

In golf, you address the ball, meaning you are in position and prepared to hit. At this point, your main concern is whether you are properly aimed at your intended target and are ready to take your shot.

In order to be mentally prepared for your swing, you run through a shot planner or pre-swing routine. There are three basic questions to ask yourself: Am I properly set up and in position? Am I properly aligned toward my target? Is my ball in the correct position? You take a minute to visualize the shot from behind the ball and perhaps choose an intermediate spot in front of the ball, in line with your primary target, to use as an alignment aid.

This is a learned process. You start out with limited knowledge and experience, but then you work hard and practice until you develop your shot plan, swing, muscle memory, and abilities. As a result, you are able to visualize your shot; you can approach the tee with confidence. You have the attitude of a winner, and everyone can sense it. You have adopted the motto "learn to improve" and taken it to heart.

Make visualization part of your daily routine and your lifestyle. What is your vision?

Thoughts on developing an originality complex

Now take this one step further and add some originality to the mix. You have contemplated and interpreted, and now you have a vision. What does it look like, feel like, taste like?

What do you intend to achieve? Perhaps it is one of the following:

---

o You want to change a negative belief, to upgrade from self-doubt to confidence. Instead of focusing on and reliving perceived failures, focus on your successes and achievements, and look forward to more.

o You want to meet the love of your life. You know you need to put yourself out there to find someone with similar wants, needs, and perspectives.

o You want to challenge yourself with a physical endurance quest. Perhaps you want to climb Mount Everest or compete in an Ironman race.

o You want to expand and develop your career, perhaps get a promotion or start a business.

How is what you propose to do different from what everyone else is doing? What is unique about your idea or approach, specifically? You want to be perceived as the only one who can do what you do, and that begins with believing in yourself.

You need to win yourself over before you can win anyone else over, so make your visualization your own. It may start out so general that it could be anyone's vision. You should end up with a vision that is distinctly your own.

You should be able to verbalize your vision in a creative and distinct way. Talk about it with friends, family, and colleagues. You are not necessarily trying to recruit a posse (unless your vision calls for that), but you are looking for a positive reaction and some constructive feedback. You want to be able to sum up your vision effectively and pitch it in such a way that you not only hold your audience's attention but you leave them wanting more. At that point, you will know you have created a tangible verbal pitch for your quest.

Your verbal pitch will then work in tandem to facilitate and support your mental vision. Having morphed and crystallized into something real that you can talk about, your vision, now easily comprehended by others, can act as a switch to allow you to jump into full visualization mode, fully engaged and in pursuit of your goal.

Now that the words and imagery are solidly in place for your vision, think about creating a TAG line for yourself. Think of TAG in this manner:

T – Thought and Talk: Contemplate and verbally define what you want to achieve.

A – Achieve: What do you hope to achieve or gain? ROI usually means Return On Investment; in this case, it can mean the Rewards Of Imagery.

You want your efforts to pay off. It's important to keep this focus in your mind and your vision.

G – Greatness: Success! Rejoice, relive, and do it again!

In the golf world, this could be your swing thought. Some of the best TAG lines have come from companies pitching products and concepts reflected in their products, a way to feel about their products, or even the desire for lifestyles supported by their products. One clear example of a successful TAG line is Nike's very clever *Just Do It* slogan. I liken it to this book's *No Excuses* TAG, and I hope you will manifest your own version of it to guide your vision of success.

Exercises to hone your visualization process

To start the visualization process, imagine yourself playing with your new golf swing; picture all the intricacies from grip to stance to alignment and the motion of flawless execution. Imagine how you look and feel as this is happening, and save this mental image of yourself for reference.

Every morning, replay your visualization in your mind. It can be a single image or moving clip of you taking your new swing in perfect form. Now think of how you feel at that moment. You are confident! You have mastered a new technique.

Perhaps you can run through this process at night as well, when you're ready for bed, so it remains in your mind as you drift off to sleep. You could even have training tools strategically placed throughout your house. For example, a friend of mine, a scratch golfer, keeps a weighted swing club in his garage. Every time he goes into the garage, it's there in plain sight, so he grabs it, does twenty or thirty relaxed swings, and then continues on. This simple action reinforces his mental visualization and keeps it fresh in his conscious mind. The ability to visualize and use mental imagery in order to maintain focus is extremely powerful.

To continue with the concept of visualization and having one main focus for your day, the idea of creating a brand new you on the golf course is reinforced when you create a brand new, improved swing. The first thing you think of in the morning and the last thing you think of at night will be that focus—your mental image of the new, improved swing coupled with physical reinforcement throughout the day when possible.

From a golf standpoint, you need to do your homework; you need to know exactly what you're dealing with. Which parts of your game need improvement? Do you honestly acknowledge your weaknesses and then strategize on how you can improve? Perhaps you can visualize because you know what is required, but you are still having difficulty making the right shots. You aren't quite focused. So what are you doing right and what are you doing wrong?

The quickest and easiest way to figure this out is to create a personal scorecard where you record the fairways hit, greens in regulation, putts, and other pieces of vital information important to your game. You are looking for patterns. You may be well aware of some, and others may come as a complete surprise. After analyzing the patterns from the scorecards you keep, you can start to develop a game-improvement program, a game plan. This should detail how you visualize your improvement, how you can improve right now, how you can physically practice, and what your improvement goals are for the next month, year, decade. You need tangible short and long term goals, and you need to be able to track your progress.

Visualization from the inside out

Our thoughts are powerful. They can become the ideas that change the world. They can invoke feelings that alter the course of our lives. They can instill a sense of what we need and want and guide us continually. Positive, progressive thought is what we need to strive for.

And here is something else worth noting: each of us has an automatic visual mechanism. It switches on and off as required. Let's say you are stretching after a strenuous workout. Your body is limber but exhausted. You try to relax and cool down on the floor mat, but your heart is still pounding, pounding. So you stop focusing on your labored breathing and start to focus on the beat of your heart—its rhythm, tone, and sensation deep within your chest. In no time at all your breathing has calmed and relaxation has won you over. Your mind and body are one.

Here is another example. One year in my vocal training, our instructor realized one of my fellow students had incredible range, and he was anxious to test her limits. He asked her to sing the scales repeatedly, each time pushing her to go a bit farther. As her vocal cords warmed up, she was able to do it, adding two or three more notes to her range. All of a sudden she broke out in laughter—she was amazed at the change and couldn't believe her own ears.

The instructor wasn't finished, though. He asked her to bring her chair to the front of the class, where she was to sing the scale again, and when she got to the note that was just out of her range she was to quickly sit down.

As we all looked at one another in anticipation, she began. As instructed, she sat down after attempting to reach the note she had missed just moments earlier. This time she hit it. They repeated the process a few more times, always striving to reach that next note, the one higher up on the scale, that previously had been out of reach.

The mental visualization drill meets TAG

To develop your visualization skills, create a daily TAG drill. First, recite your tag line. Then follow the steps below.

T – Thought and Talk: I want to successfully become the face of my business. I want to use positive internal dialogue and mental imagery so I can be effective in my approach. *I will hit that high note, the one I have never been able to reach before, and I will reach it with even tone and perfect pitch.*

A – Achieve: My achievement will be to clearly identify my core audience. They will have a sense of who I am as a representative of my business and also as a person. They will feel and react in a positive way.

G – Greatness: I'll succeed if I can convey my intentions to my audience in a manner that encourages trust.

1. Choose a scenario that best reflects your intentions and goals; for example, you may want to be a successful sales rep, keynote

speaker, or entrepreneur. Know what this looks like and feels like. How do you want others to feel about you? Respectful? Confident? Reassured? Generally your intention may be to be successful at whatever you do, and to feel important and loved.

2. Identify the detail now. In your vision, are you well dressed? Are you in a beautiful office in a modern business complex? What is the vision of your success? Consider every last detail.

3. Now close your eyes, relax, and repeat your visualization several times.

When you effectively manage your golf game, you make course management and mental techniques work to your advantage. You play smart, you trust your swing, and you work to upgrade your performance level. The same is true in your personal and work life. Both are about knowing the nature of the role required of you. By effectively visualizing yourself being successful as part of a daily drill, you will develop a mental edge. It takes time but it works.

Visualization engages the mind and encourages the body

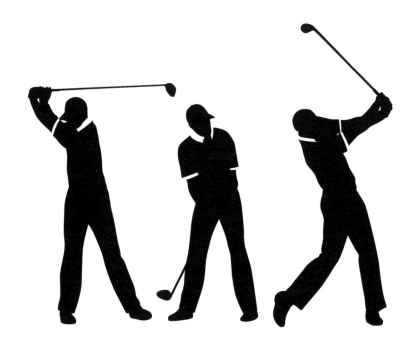

Course Management

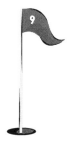

The 9th Hole – **Master Strategy**

I like to ask people, "What's your favorite time of your life so far?" The answers vary, from the dreamy-eyed glory days to a major event like buying their first house, marriage or the birth of a child, or when experiencing a high level of accomplishment and success.

Sometimes it's a fork in the road, and a drastic decision is necessary. Sometimes it's when change becomes tumultuous, even surreal. Sometimes that change can mean a glorious, unexpected adventure full of new and exciting experiences.

I suppose I would like to hear an answer like, "Right now, this is it, the very best. My life is awesome." But few of us can answer in that way, because even when we are focused and on track, eagerly chasing down success, there are often circumstantial challenges and frustrating obstacles to contend with.

And if we were ever to become completely content in life, we would no longer have to strive to exceed our expectations. Everything would remain static. And where's the fun in that?

Demystify the operatives

If you want to be a doer instead of a watcher, you need to strategize. One of the first places to start when considering a new tact or strategy is to look at what others are doing. In business, this may refer to the competition or perhaps someone whom you would consider as a mentor. Either way, ask yourself the following questions:

o How are they performing? What are their strong points, weaknesses?

o How would you compare yourself or your company to them or their company?

o What are the gaps in your competencies, directives, and expectations?

o What will it ultimately take to close those gaps?

Working with the wind

Wind can be disruptive to a game of golf, but not if you know how to work with it. Play the wind currents—crosswinds, headwinds and tailwinds—to your benefit when you can. If the wind is behind you, you may be able to "ride" it and get more distance.

If you are hitting into the wind, play the ball back in your stance, keep the trajectory low, and decrease the power of your shot by about twenty percent. Keep the ball out of the wind and in control and minimize the wind's negative impact.

When the wind is at your back, however, you may be able to capitalize on its impact in a positive way by adding yardage to your shot.

When you know what you are up against and how to deal with it, you will be able to strategically work the situation to your benefit.

Good course management or strategy in golf, business, and life dictates that you:

1. Minimize the possibility of losing momentum.

2. Maximize and capitalize on instances where there is potential for success.

Focus on where you will gain the best perspective and on those actions that will return the greatest benefits

———

One of the best strategies in life begins with combining a no-excuses mindset, a no-regrets attitude, and resilience. You then focus on building, strengthening, and reinforcing a structured, long-term plan to achieve optimal results. This is a lifestyle approach.

Once you truly master the use of a strategy and build it into a consistent, methodical process in at least one part of your life, you can adapt and alter it to work elsewhere with confidence and precision.

But first, contemplate where you can begin, where you will gain the best perspective of what you need to do to achieve your goal, and which actions will return the greatest impact.

In golf, on a par-72 course, the short-game focus usually takes priority. If you were to play a perfect game, you would take eighteen approach shots and thirty-six putts. That equates to fifty-four of seventy-two shots for 75 percent of your game. So, no excuses—if you want to improve your game rapidly, your starting point should focus on the work, exercises, and drills that will improve the most important parts of your game. Although there is not a straightforward mathematical equation to help you define your starting point for developing a life or work strategy, from a course management standpoint, this golf analogy shows you the value of doing a little up-front investigation.

Generally, you begin with a plan of action or a policy designed to achieve your overall goal. If your goal is personal in nature, you may begin by reviewing your personal traits and how you can strengthen your thought processes in order to strengthen your opportunities to achieve your goals.

Imagine a sliding scale with a low end, a high end, and a middle range. Now consider a freely moving indicator that gauges your current level, teetering back and forth in the mid-range. Where are you on the scale? What is the most efficient route from low and high? What strategy will you use to tip the scale in your favor?

What is the conversion process from low to high, and how can you apply the BIG (Brainstorm, Interpret, Go) push method to isolate your focus, own it, and increase your odds of success?

The Low End:	The High End:
Avoidance	Pursuit
Failure	Success
Anxiety	Confidence
Distress	Triumph
Immobility	Wanderlust
Low self-worth	Direction
Limitation	Vision
Excuses	Awareness

The five-stage strategy walk-through

1. **The auto-aspire phase** (*auto-aspire* is a mode of operation or way of thinking; it's when you apply the sense of becoming limitless to your life, block excuses with winning habits, and then are open to exploring the possibilities before you):

   o Evaluate performance with a focus on what you want to achieve, using a limitless aerial perspective.

   o Identify performance objectives on various levels: you independently, you as part of a team, or you and your team acting as a corporation.

   o Determine the current level of performance and the level of performance you aspire to achieve.

   o Analyze and calculate the performance gap.

2. **The expectations and being proactive phase:**

   o Convert aspirations into expectations using a proactive and dynamic plan of action. Identify critical success factors.

o Manage excuses to develop winning habits so that you are mentally prepared for success.

o Determine your BIG push strategy to advance beyond preconceived limitations.

o Draft a timeline to ensure continual forward motion toward set targets.

3. **The motivation and incentive phase:**

o Devise a strategy to effectively change behavior for yourself, your team, or your corporation.

o Consider motivation and the inclusion of an incentive plan to measure step-by-step benchmarks.

o Integrate opportunity for positive behavioral changes into daily productivity. Consider attitudes, camaraderie, and commitment.

o Validate success through acknowledgment and incentives over the life of the project.

4. **The visualize and commit phase:**

o Document and communicate projected return on investment in a succinct visual format utilizing TAG visualization.

o Identify additional areas for consideration as they relate to your current strategy.

o Encourage the prospect of continuing development and commitment to growth and improvement.

o Award individuals for their achievements in the success of the overall strategy. Create a challenge to encourage others to follow suit.

5. **The formulate-a-curriculum phase** (write down your course of action):

o Be credible by clearly documenting the No Excuses Success Action Plan details.

o Identify the aspiration, the expectation, and the gap that needs to be filled.

o Identify the opportunity, the motivation, the incentive, and the desired outcome.

o Detail results as you progress.

Master strategy? Self-regulation, coaching, and mentorship

You know you've got some game in you. You want to prove it to yourself, and perhaps you want to prove it to the world. Striving to attain peak performance, practicing and honing endurance and push drills, developing effective course management, and ridding yourself of excuses are all strategies you can develop to stack the odds of success in your favor. These strategies are what take you to the next level by building on the concepts we have been exploring so far in this book. Think of your strategy as a form of coaching in which the goal is a high level of individual and/or team efficacy whereby achievement is a given. No excuses, regrets, or roadblocks!

If you are intending to use the assistance of a coach or mentor to achieve your goals, consider that the measure of effective coaching involves three key strategic functions:

1. to provide instruction

2. to oversee the practice of required skills

3. to offer consistent, constructive feedback

Moreover, success in coaching is directly tied to the quality of the coach/protégé relationship as it builds over time. Following are the key ingredients crucial to coaching success.

The BREADTH of coaching/mentoring strategy

———

I use this acronym to detail the relationship dynamics as they relate to the coaching/mentoring strategy.

B - Belief: The expectations of the relationship. The coach believes in the talents and abilities of the protégé, and the protégé believes the coach will be able to push her to perform at an optimal level she may not be able to attain on her own.

R - Respect: The value of the relationship. Both the coach and protégé feel confident that they will both give exceptional focus to what is required and what is being achieved.

E - Engagement: The nature of the relationship. The coach and protégé collectively work to build and sustain a healthful, constructive interaction. Reciprocity is a given. There is a constant desire to help each other because they are genuinely interested in achieving a common goal.

A - Advocacy: The voice of the relationship. The coach and protégé aim for real camaraderie and desire to achieve predefined goals.

D - Determination: The momentum of the relationship. The coach facilitates the protégé's progress by minimizing distraction, providing guidance, downplaying failure, and up-playing successes to establish and reinforce continual forward motion toward a goal.

T - Trust: The integrity of the relationship. The coach trusts that she is receiving 100 percent of the protégé's efforts, and the protégé trusts that the coach is competent and committed to the project.

H - Heart: The level of soul within the relationship. Both coach and protégé are eager to push beyond their limits and as a result feel a great investment toward the end result—the win.

As you analyze and decipher the aspects of coaching effectiveness, it becomes clear just how important a good working relationship can be to the overall success of your strategy. When you apply the systematic and achievement oriented objectives of coaching/mentoring to self-regulation, solid working strategies develop, and the overall process changes to a more succinct and direct approach. Design the process to be acted upon, develop a monitoring system to oversee efficient execution of the plan, gather constructive feedback, and use it to improve and redefine the process.

The BREADTH self-coaching message: believe in yourself!

If you are intending to pursue your goals on your own, consider applying the BREADTH approach to a personal self-coaching strategy. It really isn't that different as long as you take your achievements seriously. You may not have the camaraderie and relationship in place, but you can still apply all of the same tactics as outlined in BREADTH by remaining consistent, constructive and most importantly, by believing in yourself!

Believe...
that you are the only one who can do what you do in the way that you do it!

Congratulations!

You've just finished your front nine! In the front nine, we've dealt with the basics of using peak performance strategies to achieve optimal results by converting aspirations into expectations and excuses into winning habits. These strategies include becoming limitless, taking an aerial perspective, creating and developing aspirations, managing excuses, pushing to stay proactive, and honing your motivational and strategic skills. These strategies will work in tandem with an incentive plan to attain your goals and fulfill your vision.

When you use course management as your guide, you have peak performance skills at your fingertips. You've sharpened your attitude and motivation to achieve your goals. Now, armed with solid visualization strategies geared toward success, you are ready to support a No Excuses Success Action Plan and the lifestyle that will follow.

That means you're ready for the back nine, where the focus is on putting all the front nine's basics into play, whether in the workplace or your personal pursuit of success.

At the Turn:
Advance the Ball

In golf, when you finish your front nine, you are "at the turn." It's the time to take a breather, grab a refreshment, and then get started on the back nine.

So far, I've been talking about working the mind-body-achievement connection and the components of a success action plan for peak performance. Now, for your breather, I want you to reflect on what you want out of your personal and work life.

In golf, you want every shot to advance the ball closer to your intended target. The most efficient route is the winning route.

In the front nine, as we progressed hole by hole, we were advancing the ball. Each chapter introduced and developed a new concept to tweak your mental prowess and prepare you for the back nine: The Lifestyle Prototype.

To recap:

The 1st Hole – Be limitless: Becoming limitless involves training to be mentally and physically poised, with your mind and body working in harmony to achieve a successful outcome. It means going after and getting what you want.

The 2nd Hole – The aerial perspective: Stay focused on an objective overview of your goal. Stick to the facts and strip out emotion as you think. If you start to question or doubt anything about yourself or your goal, stop. Refocus specifically on the high-level goal only—its value and its merit.

The 3rd Hole – Aspirations: The promise of aspiration is that it is evolutionary. The human condition is such that we are always aspiring to be something more, something better, something nobler. It starts as a thought, a want, a need, or a desire and then grows and evolves with intention and direction, sometimes with lust and hunger. The continued drive feeds the rise.

The 4th Hole – Excuse management: When you actively take measures to manage what is controllable in your life, you'll find that you stop making excuses. Fully engaged and strategically focused on your intended target, you drive your ball toward the best possible outcome—and you forget about making excuses. It may not be your final destination, but at least you are in control and out of excuse-making mode.

The 5th Hole – The BIG push: The BIG push means being able to develop and sustain momentum toward your goal; it is the process of actively replacing excuses with winning habits, the ultimate excuse blockers. Moreover, it is being willing to go to the wall for what you want or believe in, to push beyond your previous mental and physical limits, no matter what it takes.

The 6th Hole – Motivation: Motivation is the force that initiates, guides, and sustains our achievement-oriented behavior over time. It is what causes us to take action, be willing to commit, and stick with our goals even when we experience setbacks.

The 7th Hole – Inspiration and incentive: Incentives work well when they are properly structured, monitored, and administered. They must be realistic, attainable, and of benefit either singularly or mutually to those involved. If an incentive plan is layered over an effective action-oriented strategy, it will reinforce the force and flow of the strategy. There needs to be opportunity, inspiration, motivation, incentive, and ultimately knowledge that the outcome is attainable.

The 8th Hole – The vision: Visualization is a creative effort. You imagine and cultivate every detail about something you want to achieve to create lasting mental pictures of yourself achieving your goals or improving your performance. When you imagine yourself achieving something, your brain will work to find a way to make it happen. It is like a mental rehearsal for success.

The 9th Hole – The master strategy: One of the best strategies in life begins with combining a no-excuses mindset, a no-regrets attitude, and resilience. You then focus on building, strengthening, and reinforcing a structured, long-term plan to achieve optimal results. This is a lifestyle approach.

Once you truly master the use of a strategy and build it into a consistent, methodical process in at least one part of your life, you can adapt and alter it to work elsewhere with confidence and precision.

I was recently asked, "When do you stop focusing on what you want to achieve?" The answer: not until after you have decided to believe in yourself, successfully achieved your goal, and have moved on to your next goal. Hold your successes close and relive the thrill of the win again and again and again.

For every forward action, there is an equally important forward reaction

In the historic days of war, the winning army would pillage and loot the conquered countryside. These newly acquired possessions were considered the spoils of victory. Today that term is used more metaphorically. When you achieve your goals in life, in addition to the win that you've been focused on, there are peripheral spoils to claim. Aside from the literal win, you gain the benefits that go with the win—status, opportunity, and perks. Your confidence grows, you feel better, you think more clearly, and you believe in the power of you!

Ad victorem spolias
To the victor, the spoils
—Anonymous

The Back Nine:
The Lifestyle Prototype

Visualize the Shot

In the front nine, we dealt with various attitudes and strategies you need to adopt in order to be successful. In this section, I want you to use the course management approach to create a working success action plan coupled with solid visualization techniques to create a health and fitness lifestyle prototype.

This section, the back nine, can almost be viewed as a separate book. I hope that you continue on and take the challenge to actively work through these holes (chapters). This is where you have the opportunity to build the success action strategies we have discussed, adopting them in your day-to-day life to create winning habits and building strategies for competitive play.

To put that action plan into play, the following nine chapters will reintroduce concepts from the front nine in detail, including a solid working example, and explore what it takes to build a fit, healthy, and strong lifestyle. This will be a visual expression of confidence, your personal body brand, and the resulting lifestyle prototype. Consider the prospect of exercising your mind and body in a new way, in tandem, to reap the benefit of the mind-body-achievement connection.

You will learn that the winners in life not only see the big picture, but they imagine the role they will play and they visualize how they will make their success action plans and strategies work. They break big-picture stuff into smaller pieces so they can attack and deal with them one by one. They build skills, knowledge, self-esteem, and whatever they need so they are ready to compete and face challenges.

Visualizing the shot involves using the power of imagination. You imagine your best shot as you stand behind the ball, using a mental picture that clearly paints an imaginary line from where you are standing to where you want your ball to come to rest. Once you get good at this, it is an incredible tool.

I sometimes visualize myself in a practice swing. I pull smoothly into my backswing and stop, and I mentally check my grip, my form, my stance. I ask myself, "Am I ready to take the shot?"

The value of using your imagination cannot be overestimated. Excitement and enthusiasm is created when your thoughts are so heightened and focused that your mind connects your thoughts, emotions, and body with actual physical outcomes.

If you don't recognize your imagination and use it, you're not using all of your tools to be successful. Your performance strategy plan needs to start with imagery: seeing what needs to happen and seeing how you're going to make it happen.

Life itself is the most intense, most strategized game there is, so let's look at how to approach this game by getting you set up and aligned so that you are aimed properly at your intended target. That's what these last nine holes are all about—breaking down the big picture to achieve optimal results, being able to visualize the shot, understanding all of the details and intricacies of what is required to make the shot, and being ready to win.

Just as you did with the front nine, in the back nine, you need to design and build your own positive mental image, one that will allow you to see how to take charge of your life and envision the physical outcome you desire. Then, most importantly, you have to take action.

Swing Thoughts:

Decide to accept challenge.

Develop winning habits and visualization techniques.

Climb the leader board (a scoreboard showing the top performers in a competition, particularly a golf tournament).

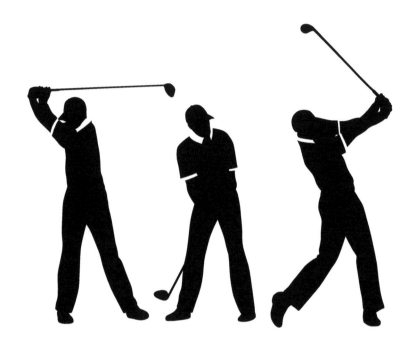

Visualize the Shot

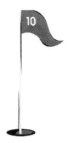

The 10th Hole – **Strategy Phase I:**

Auto-aspire

It's crucial to awaken the explorer within you, your inner kid, the part of you that is adventurous, inquisitive, and perhaps a little impetuous. You can do this by engaging in what I call "auto-aspire" mode, which is when you apply the sense of becoming limitless to your life. You block excuses with winning habits, and you then examine the possibilities before you. You do this often, until it becomes second nature, or automatic.

Not all aspirations will come to fruition. But most of them deserve to be explored, and functioning in auto-aspire mode enables this process. You act to raise your subconscious level to the extent that being open to exploring your aspirations becomes automatic for you. This will require you to repeatedly ask yourself very pointed questions until these questions become part of your mindful daily routine.

To effectively function in full auto-aspire mode, you need to open your mind and become intuitively aware of your thoughts and feelings, your authentic self—*not* the adult, the always-in-control you that you present to the world day after day.

So dig down deep into your awareness and honestly answer the following questions:

o   Where do I go from here?

o   If I were to open my mind, what opportunities would there be for me?

o   What can I achieve and how much time do I need to invest?

o   Does this make sense for me?

o   What have I always wanted to do?

o   Have I erected roadblocks to stifle my potential? If so, how can I break them down?

You are limitless, boundless, and inexhaustible

In the introduction, I discussed the three top goals people target yet fail to achieve—losing weight, getting in shape, and becoming healthier overall. This is where excuses most commonly build up, causing willpower to falter and failure to prevail. On the back nine, we are going to address these three issues. We will learn to replace excuses with winning habits by tackling a no-excuses challenge coupled with a fitness challenge.

In the front nine, you learned how to identify and crush excuses, and now you need to take action. That's what creating a working lifestyle prototype in the back nine is all about. We can all improve in one way or another. Continual improvement and relevant forward motion gravitating toward your goal is the key to your success.

When we delve deeper, it becomes apparent that to achieve any such high-concept quests, it is crucial to establish a meaningful sense of self-worth and self-confidence, acknowledge known talents, and develop psychological skills. This is where the mind-body-achievement connection comes into play. It is the honed ability to become and stay motivated, provide yourself with incentives, and push your mind and body into high-functioning achievement mode. All your aerial perspective quests will benefit from the combination of mental and physical strategies.

The evolution of the mind-body-achievement connection, from an aerial perspective, is where the power behind the process begins. To recap, it is the following peak performance strategies that will empower you and enable you to develop and work through the SAP for any target you may choose.

Peak performance highlights:

o Develop the mentality of a contender. Believe in your ability to achieve!

o Keep your target in sight or mind at all times. Learn to effectively TAG and visualize your quest.

o Be determined. Don't let excuses drag you sideways. Develop winning habits.

o Encourage and reward successes. If you give up, you reward failure.

o Plan for the weak moments. To maintain momentum, you need to be able to recover quickly.

If your mind and body are working in unison, you can achieve great things in your life. Your body will be strong and resilient, and as a result, you will feel confident, fit, and in control.

Your healthy body will fuel your brain and keep your mind sharp. You will be able to focus, adapt, and realign as required. You won't get lost or sidetracked by unimportant factors or excuses along the way.

Maintaining a healthy mind and body is tantamount to achieving success in life. Almost everything of importance that you tackle will require continued staying power and stick-to-itiveness—over the long haul, you have to stay the course.

Promote insight and raise consciousness

Here is an observation. Say you run into some friends or colleagues you haven't seen for a while, and you begin a conversation. You catch up for a couple of moments, but then what do you talk about? Is it new, interesting stuff or the same-old, same-old, regurgitated stuff?

I talk to a lot of people in the course of a day, and I almost always gravitate to those whom I know will have something interesting to say. I know I am not the only one who thinks this way.

What characteristics do you seek out in those around you? Is it a spark? A certain energy and excitement? Is it being tempted and tantalized so you can't wait to respond, "Yes, that's it! I understand. I get you!" When we talk to others who have fresh thoughts and ideas and a lot to say, we are interested and tend to gravitate to them. We want to hear what they have to say.

What renders these folks interesting? They have learned how to function in auto-aspire mode. They are always aspiring, to the point that it becomes automatic and subconscious. They begin every morning on the right side. They are eagerly in search of new opportunities, and they do not limit the scope of their reality. They believe that today is the beginning of something great. And the most exciting aspect of thinking this way is that anyone can do it if they so choose.

Shake out some aspirational moxie— this is how you do it!

I like to surround myself with bold statements. As a writer, I love words, their impact, and their appeal. TAGs and swing thoughts should all be as bold as you can dream up. Here are some examples of bold statements you can you use every morning to gear up for auto-aspire mode.

o I want to be fit, healthy, and strong.

o I know that how I look and act is a visual expression of my confidence.

o I know that my attitude and appearance defines my personal brand.

o I am going to develop a strong mind, sleek physique and optimal health to reinforce the mind-body-achievement connection.

How about this bold statement:

> Obesity is a leading cause of preventable illness and death in North America. In recent years, the number of overweight people in industrialized countries has increased significantly, so much so that the World Health Organization (WHO) has called obesity an epidemic. In the United States, over 65 percent of the adult population is overweight. In Canada, about 40 percent to 60 percent of adults have a weight problem.

> People who are obese are at a much higher risk for serious medical conditions such as high blood pressure, heart attack, stroke, diabetes, gallbladder disease, and different cancers than people who have a healthy weight. (Source: http://bodyandhealth. canada.com/condition_info_details. asp?disease_id=95)

In other words, your health is your responsibility. No excuses!

Most of us, at one time or another, have decided that it was absolutely time to get in shape. For whatever reason, we pick a date and make a resolution to lose weight, workout, and eat more healthily. And how great would it be to be able to say, "This time *I did it!*"

Take time to fill out the following summary before moving on to the next chapter. For these exercises, I use weight loss as an example, and I give you a sample answer for each. Fill in with your own goals.

The Lifestyle Prototype

The Auto-Aspire Phase Summary:

1. Evaluate your performance with a focus on what you want to achieve, using a limitless aerial perspective.

   ☞ I am in moderate shape, probably ten to fifteen pounds overweight.

   ☞ _____

   ☞ _____

2. Identify performance objectives on various levels: You independently, you as part of a team, or you and your friends or colleagues acting as a team.

   ☞ I am going to lose weight, get in shape, and become healthier overall.

   ☞ _____

   ☞ _____

3. Determine your current level of performance and the level of performance you aspire to achieve.

   ☞ I am going to make positive changes in my life. I am going to establish a routine and stick with it. I am going to continue to work hard at achieving my goals until my efforts become automatic in nature.

   ☞ _____

   ☞ _____

4. Interpret and calculate your performance gap.

   ☞ To achieve my goal, I need to do cardio and weight training, clean up my diet, and become healthier overall. I am making a lifestyle overhaul.

☞ _____.

☞ _____.

Live your life on auto-aspire.
Aspire to regular good habits that become
automatic and second nature.

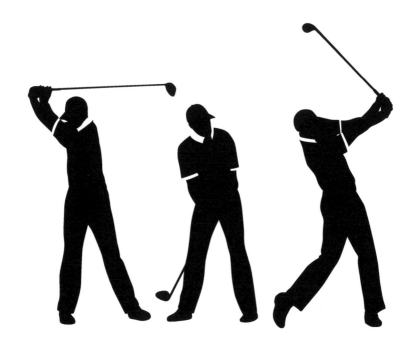

Visualize the Shot

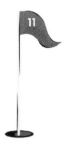

The 11th Hole – **Strategy Phase II:**

Expectations and Being Proactive

It is not enough to accept a challenge and expect to learn, change, improve, and achieve. You need to take what you have learned and proactively put it into play. That is exactly what we are looking at on this hole.

From the auto-aspire phase and exercises, your performance evaluation and aspirational brainstorming should have churned out some solid, hard-core directives for you—those blanks you filled in in the exercises. Now you are going to back them up with some substance. In this chapter, you'll move away from the free-form exploratory mode of auto-aspire to a more regimented mode. You want to define your expectations. You want to ensure that your expectations are realistic, achievable, and in line with your beliefs. You want to know that the aspirations that you decide to pursue will eventually lead you where you want to go. At that point, you can truly expect to achieve your goals. There will be no more *maybe*, *hopefully*, or *perhaps* word blocks, just a clear expectation of a specific outcome.

Being proactive defines your ability to achieve

Let's revisit the BIG push from the 5th Hole chapter, where being proactive was defined as the decision made to initiate positive change on an ongoing basis. You want to replace excuses with winning habits in a dramatic way, to go after what you want or what you believe in, to push beyond your mental and physical limits, and to go for whatever you want in life no matter what it takes.

Here is my take again on winning habits. Commit to a minimum of sixty hours, equally spread over a ten week period of your life, push your positive routines and activities to the winning-habit level, and change your life forever. When you get to the point where you automatically summon positive responses to any problem or challenge, you will have reached the auto-aspire stage and upgraded to living life in the no-excuses zone.

Change what you can change

There are things you can't change and there are things you shouldn't change. For instance, you cannot change the past; you can only change how you think and feel about it. You can learn from it and use that information moving forward. Things you shouldn't attempt to change? Don't waste time on concepts, products or beliefs that are of no viable use to you in your quest for self-improvement and growth.

I mention this to introduce the flipside, which is that if something *can* be changed, change it. Expect that there is something better to be created—a new concept, product or idea, a by-product. Use some personal creativity, and try to question why things are what they are. Quite often there is a better way of doing things. Sometimes a total reconstruct is required.

When you begin to expect that there is always room for improvement, you put yourself in the driver's seat. Why wait for someone else to figure it out or do it? Expect that you are the one. Expect great outcomes. Expect that you are the best candidate and that you will achieve your goals.

Golf is definitely a game of strategy. It offers a multilevel and seemingly limitless source of personal challenges. First, you are playing against the course, and there is a wide variety of course difficulty as defined by par for the course, the overall length, and the slope. Second, you are playing against yourself by trying to reduce your overall score and handicap. Third, you can compete against others based on your total score for eighteen holes (stroke play) or on a hole-by-hole basis (match play), where you compete with another player or team. You can also play level (straight up) or off handicap.

If I expect to become a better golfer, and I always do, I create specific expectations such as to improve my putting or to develop my accuracy with pitch shots. Then I create an action plan to proactively target improving my skills so I can meet or even exceed my expectations. I write out every important detail of the changes I want to make, clearly and concisely, so I know what I need to do and how I am going to do it.

The more challenges you accept, the more you learn and the more you become willing to take on more challenges. So now, armed with aspirations, expectations, and the gap you need to fill, ask yourself, "How can I be proactive and own 100 percent of my focus?"

What is fitness if not a series of endurance drills? The difference here is the BIG push, proactively going after what you want to achieve

Practice, practice, practice—then rest, recover, regroup, strategize, and rebound. At this point, the majority of people are focusing on the best possible outcome, and that is fine. It's positive and optimistic. But that is only part of the game plan. Always endeavor to take a different approach. Step back. Rethink and revisit your approach with a fresh perspective and unbiased attitude. For example, what is the worst situation or position you could possibly find yourself in? Train so that if you find yourself in such a situation, you will know how to fix it. You will feel positive and optimistic on a broader scale, and that is extremely important in building a confident, determined mindset.

On the golf course, whenever you have an errant shot—a shot that leaves you in long grass, under a tree, in loose and tangled brush, or in the water— you will need a recovery shot to get your ball back into play. Your recovery shot needs to be set up so you have a good lie and are in position to make your next shot. You cannot afford another wasted shot, so you expect to recover and be proactive by setting up your next shot. You know how to work a great recovery shot into your game because you have practiced these shots in anticipation of a situation like this.

When you approach your endurance drills by starting at the most difficult position you can be in, you can improve your accuracy more quickly and push yourself to the next level faster. Since you know you are starting at a more difficult level, there's no need to harshly judge your performance, and because you haven't done this before, there's no need for excuses. Set aside your repertoire of objections and own 100 percent of your focus.

Swing trigger, anyone?

A golf swing trigger is part of the pre-shot routine. It's the process of preparing to take your shot. In golf, when you go to hit the ball it is not moving. It is simply sitting there, on the ground, waiting for you to hit it. And there is silence, sometimes so much silence that it's distracting. Everyone is watching you and waiting for you, and if you dwell on this, it could spell disaster.

Thus the pre-shot routine is intended to help you deal with nerves and focus on your game. Often this routine is set in motion by the golfer by invoking a swing trigger, an act that switches the player into focus mode. An example could be putting on your glove, stretching, or even taking a deep, relaxing breath. Think about how you could use a trigger to help you with your focus.

Push hard and expect rapid results

Here are some proactive mantras that I have developed over the years:

o   Don't expect to be perfect, but work hard nonetheless.

- o Don't be tempted to break momentum—work through it.

- o Don't hesitate and second-guess yourself. Just be the best you can be in every step you take toward your goal.

- o Don't compromise your focus by comparing what you are trying to learn to what you already know. Focus in the moment, on what you are trying to learn now.

- o Own 100 percent of your focus. The most challenging of endurance drills will bring you to a level of optimal mental and physical performance.

Which one(s) do you relate to? Do you have your own to add to the list?

The BIG push falls in behind taking your authentic aspirations, filling any knowledge or skills gap, tying expectations to your aspirations, and then pushing beyond what is generally accepted as average.

If you wanted to be average, you would not be reading this book

So what can you do—right now?

You know what you want to achieve, and you believe and expect that you can achieve it. You are also very aware of excuses that may come into play, and with them in mind you commit to forging ahead using positive winning-habit routines and activities. You develop and perfect endurance drills, push yourself every day, and ultimately own 100 percent of your focus. You know that if something is changeable, you have as much opportunity to make that change as the next person.

Keeping the lifestyle prototype in mind, your expectations will be fitness and health oriented. Consider your top three aspirations and how you would go about converting them into expectations. What form of action would you take to ensure success and how would you go about it? Think proactively and dynamically. Be realistic, but set your sights high.

What do you want to accomplish today, this week, this month, or this year?

Looking to take your success to the next level? Upgrade your skills. Build winning habits. Proactively do the work!

Here are some examples to get into the right frame of mind:

Build enduring, healthful, "feel good" habits:

Current State: I am out of shape and don't feel good about myself.

Aspiration/Goal: To lose weight, work out, get in shape, and feel better mentally and physically.

Expectations: I will walk two miles every day and clean up my eating habits for at least ten weeks.

Build willpower to overpower unhealthful behavior:

Current State: I am sluggish and out of breath. I got the memo—I know how bad smoking is for me and I want to quit, but I am struggling and frustrated.

Aspiration/Goal: To quit smoking for good.

Expectations: I will consult my doctor, get on a quit-smoking program, and make a positive lifestyle change.

Build healthful, competitive achievement strategies:

Current State: I have always been a fairly good athlete, but I have never pushed myself to really excel at any one thing.

Aspiration/Goal: To build my fitness and endurance prowess and win a competition.

Expectations: I am going to get a trainer, commit to a healthful lifestyle that supports my efforts, and sign up for the Ironman competition next year.

Build confidence and replace my excuses with winning habits:

Current State: I am in a rut, repeating the same mistakes and standing still.

Aspiration/Goal: To take on small challenges and gradually build the skills required to effectively tackle larger goals.

Expectations: I am going take hold of my life, both mentally and physically. I am going to gag my inner critic and listen to and embrace my inner cheerleader. I am going to lean on my mentor and support team and work hard to transform my life.

Build my body awareness with some "me" time:

Current State: I am tired of being tired and rushing through life.

Aspiration/Goal: To honor my body, reduce stress, and sharpen my thought processes.

Expectations: I am going to improve my eating habits, exercise, learn to relax, and invest in some time-management training.

Complete the following summary before proceeding to the next chapter. For these exercises, weight loss is again used as an example. A sample answer is provided for each. Fill in with your own targets.

The Lifestyle Prototype

The Expectations and Being Proactive Phase Summary:

1. Convert aspirations into expectations using a proactive and dynamic plan of action. Identify critical success factors.

   ☞ I am going to lose weight, get in shape, and become healthier overall by following a detailed FIT program. I will start with a physical so I can identify where I need to improve, then take my measurements so I can calculate real change.

   ☞ _____

   ☞ _____

2. Implement excuse management to develop winning habits so that you are mentally prepared for success.

↦ I am going to create a workout schedule and healthful food plan and stick to it for a minimum of ten weeks. This is where I have failed in the past; I deviated from my plan and lost interest. I have fallen into the bad habit of making excuses for why I don't stick to my plan. I am now very aware of how excuses have eroded my ability to achieve in the past, and this time I am focusing on winning habits so I don't cave in under pressure. This time I am expecting great outcomes.

↦ _____

↦ _____

3. Determine BIG push strategy to advance beyond preconceived limitations.

↦ I will monitor my progress, paying particular attention to slipping into a stall phase. Whenever I feel that my progress has slowed, I will push harder by upgrading my workout strategy or altering my routine. I may even push to exhaustion from time to time. I want results.

☞ _____

☞ _____

4. Create a timeline to ensure continual forward motion toward set targets.

☞ I have settled on a ten-week program for now. I will take my starting point, a list of key factors like weight and measurements, perhaps blood pressure and cholesterol level, and then I will identify realistic and attainable targets for the end of week ten. I will then split the total change I wish to make into ten chunks or benchmarks. Ten weeks to winning habits. Ten weeks to a new and improved me! Each week I will be able to compare my actual performance with the change I had planned and expected.

☞ _____

☞ _____

Expectations are made to be exceeded!

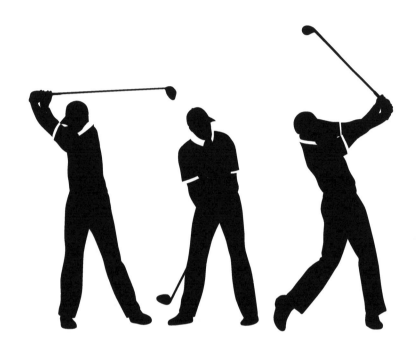

Visualize the Shot

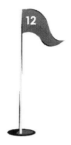

The 12ᵗʰ Hole – **Strategy Phase III:**

Motivation and Incentives

Most of us are continually engaged in some form of pursuit. We are seeking excellence within one or more areas in our lives, and that is the basis of our motivation. It is human nature to have a *need* to get ahead, to need a little something more—it's in our DNA. Although we may not be certain of what we need at any given moment, we know there's something. It's a competitive itch and desire to improve that never goes away.

Thus, if you are like most people, you're moderately driven. You are successfully moving through life, building relationships, achieving things, pushing yourself to excel, and enjoying the ride. Life is generally good.

But what if you could boost your motivation to a "totally driven" level? What would life be like

---

then? Would you become more aspirational, entertain a higher level of expectation for yourself, feel more engaged, and be more motivated to get up every morning ready to take on the world, kick some ass, and rejoice in the splendor of your brilliance?

While functioning at this level could be quite exhausting, not only for you but for everyone around you, knowing and understanding your motivation is critical. You will be most effective when you have identified your motivation and believe that it holds value for you.

A show of confidence raises the bar

When you take your achievements, one by one, no matter what their independent value, and stack them, one by one, you continue to build their overall impact; together small changes and improvements add up. Here is an example:

Current State: I am a weekend warrior, meaning I don't make time to improve my sport, I just run out at the last minute to sneak a golf game in and hope to play well—and usually don't.

Aspiration/Goal: To be a better golfer.

Expectations: I will retool my exercise regimen to develop the strength, flexibility, and endurance

I need to improve my game. I will hit the driving range and work to improve my accuracy, and I will commit to playing golf once a week.

Do I want this? Yes! Is there value for me? Yes! Am I going to make this happen? Yes!

You're killing me

We all covet life, and to some degree, we all carry positive thoughts, experiences, and meaning. We also carry around a lot of other stuff—quite often stuff we don't need. My question is why?

Why do you need negative thoughts, experiences, or meaning? For example, when it comes to your health, why would you tolerate huffing and puffing because you are out of shape, especially if it may be causing you harm?

What happened? How did your lifestyle change so much that you didn't take notice of the lack of activity? How did you justify the bigger clothes in your closet? Where did you hide the weigh scale? Where did your motivation go? It may have happened too gradually to even have been noticed, but at some point the excuses must stop.

Imagine a bright red balloon filled with motivation, and MOTIVATION printed in big block letters on its surface, floating gently in the air. A slow leak starts, then a tear, and before you know it the balloon is spiraling around the room, back and forth and all over before finally settling in a heap on the floor, fully deflated.

Motivation: to think myself successful!

Let's again take the example of health and fitness. What is your fitness motivation?

o I want to feel great.

o I want to build muscle and feel in control of my body.

o I want to be strong, both mentally and physically.

o I want to be fit and able to maintain that fitness level well into my senior years.

o I want to be able to perform everyday activities with ease.

o I want to defy the normal process of aging.

o I want to improve my balance and agility.

o I want to boost my stamina.

o   I want to strengthen my core.

o   I want to minimize my aches and pains.

Now ask yourself… Do I want this? Yes! Is there value for me? Yes! Am I going to make this happen? Yes!

You can reinforce your pursuit of your expectations by incorporating a personal incentive plan. Here is an example from *Targeting Success*, the first book in the *3 Off the Tee* series.

Last year, when my weight was creeping up, I threw out a little competitive challenge to a group of my friends. Golf season was coming, and we were all complaining about having gained weight over the winter. My idea was not terribly original, but it certainly worked for us.

This is the No Excuses Challenge I e-mailed to my friends:

Pre-season Tune-Up!

Here it is-the No Excuses Challenge! Sweet and simple. Lose some weight and perhaps make some cash. It all comes down to how competitive you are.

Here's how it works. First, you commit to losing ten pounds in ten weeks. Then, you pay $500 into a weight-loss fund. For every pound you lose, you earn back $50. If you lose the full ten pounds, it will have cost you nothing, but you will have lost ten pounds. At the end of the program, if you have lost your ten pounds, you will also get to split the balance of the cash not earned back by your competitors, who, for whatever reason, didn't lose their entire ten pounds.

Let's see what kind of a loser you really are!

I then asked people to e-mail me to join and each day thereafter to text or e-mail their weight to me until the final weigh-in.

Everyone who took the challenge succeeded. They each lost ten or more pounds. For some, the competition alone was enough; they kept track of everyone's weight loss, and it kept them focused. Others were motivated by their competitor's plans to spend their winnings, and there was no way they would be paying out for that to happen.

I had the least amount of weight to lose and, surprisingly, lost the last half pound by the morning of the final weigh-in. That was close! Nevertheless, I won my money back, and I lost the weight.

The interesting part of this challenge was that, when people initially read it, they felt compelled to ask me how they were supposed to lose the weight. I told them that there was no real plan. They had to figure out what would work for them and then do it. Deep down, we all know what we need to do, don't we? If we want to be healthy and look healthy, with a nice physique, pleasant appearance, and engaging manner, we need to eat right, get enough sleep, exercise, and manage stress. It's as simple as that.

For those who like a challenge, this was an irresistible proposition. Those not so inclined failed to respond or declined. This was ultimately why my challenge-loving participants succeeded. They were up for the challenge. Will you accept the same challenge and put it in place with your friends and colleagues?

You accept challenge because you enjoy it. You are competitive, usually a good sport, and perhaps you are strong and have learned to be resilient. You win—you win. You lose—you bounce back and try again. Hopefully this sounds familiar to you.

How to be up for the challenge

Resilience is not a commodity you are born with, waiting silently on tap. It is self-manufactured painstakingly over time by working through your problems and never giving up, even in the face of difficulty or failure.

The best way to build your resilience is to start with some attainable, realistic, smaller goals, and then gradually and regularly increase the volume or intensity of the challenge. I call this challenge *chunking*: bite-sized goals, once achieved, lead to big-time confidence building.

When you are honest with yourself, develop the right skills and attributes, strategize, and work hard, accepting a challenge is easy. You learn to trust your swing. Just as a healthy body fuels a healthy mind, a mind that's open to challenge is strong, resilient, and ready to win. Focus on developing the following attributes when creating chunking strategies: awareness, confidence, persistence, determination, courage, direction, curiosity, ingenuity, and creativity.

In all my books, I reach out to readers for feedback. This little challenge caught on, and I started getting letters and e-mails describing how people had accepted my challenge and how it worked for them. There were interesting variations—some substituted ten percent weight loss for the ten pounds, and some lowered the dollar value to $100. Yet the one that jumped out at me was one in which a group of guys decided to lose twenty-five pounds in six months and then keep that weight off for an additional eighteen months with regular weigh-ins at monthly intervals. The dollar amount on the line—$5,000. Now there was a competition! Was it too costly? Obviously, no one would enter such a competition without a fierce desire to win.

Implementing an incentive plan to reward positive change

Incentive plans work best when they are structured, monitored, and administered. They must be realistic, attainable (say, having twenty-five pounds to lose), and they must benefit either singularly or mutually to those involved. In my example above, everyone had the same advantages and opportunities to lose the weight and potentially win the money should their competitors fail to do so.

Consider the following:

Current State: Things are okay but I would like to make some positive, healthful changes in my life.

Aspiration/Goal: To be able to fit into and look great in fashionable clothes.

Expectations: I want to feel secure and confident. To achieve this, I know looking good, healthy, and youthful are important factors; when I feel good about how I look, I feel more secure about myself and I am not afraid of rejection.

In fact, I generally experience less anxiety and push myself harder when I feel in control of myself, which reinforces my motivation to feel secure and confident. I want to buy a new, size-reduced wardrobe and rock my high school reunion.

You want to lose weight so you will look and feel better. As an incentive (reward), you will go on a minor shopping spree when you achieve this goal. Something comes up, though—problems at work or home and then some dinners out where you fall off your diet. You become frustrated with your lack of progress in losing weight, so you decide to buy some new clothes anyhow, just to make yourself feel better. But now, you've just turned your incentive for losing weight into an incentive for not losing weight. You overturned your personal incentive plan, rendering it of no value. Don't reward failure!

Benchmarking by calories, clothing sizes, and inches

At the beginning of the No Excuses Challenge (my ten-week weight-loss plan for me and my friends), I took some time to set goals and did my usual beginning routine of taking a *before* picture and jotting down my weight and measurements at different points on my body. This always helps me to get psyched up. Weight loss really wasn't my top priority. My focus was more on making healthful choices and getting in shape.

At the end of week three, I had lost four pounds, which left me with six more to go. I then compared my new measurements with my start measurements. I kept two categories, the first for places where I wanted to lose inches and the second for places where I wanted to build muscle and thus gain inches. For me and my goals, body reshaping was as important as losing excess weight.

By benchmarking by calories, clothing sizes, and inches, I could reward myself. For example I could buy new clothes for the spring—short, sexy dresses and some sleek new golf wear.

Complete the following. As before, for these exercises, weight loss is used as an example, and you're given a sample response for each. Fill in with your own goals, whether they are on a professional or personal level.

The Lifestyle Prototype

The Motivation and Incentive Phase Summary:

1. Devise a strategy to effectively change behavior for yourself, your team, or your corporation.

☞ To eat responsibly and exercise in order to lose weight, get in shape and become healthier overall.

☞ _____

☞ _____

2. Consider your motivation levels and the inclusion of an incentive plan when looking to implement benchmarks to measure and monitor step-by-step transition.

☞ I am motivated by a fear of becoming unhealthy, which elicits a desire to feel and look better. I will reward my successes at intervals based on the benchmarks en route to my overall goal.

☞ _____

☞ _____

3. Make positive behavioral changes in your daily routine and interaction with others. Consider attitudes, camaraderie, and commitment.

☞ I will alter my daily routine to become generally more active. I will be open to helping others to make changes for themselves, and I will commit to reaching my own goals.

☞ _____

☞ _____

4. Validate your successes through acknowledgment and incentives over the life of the project.

   ☞ New clothes, spa day, personal trainer, new golf clubs?

   ☞ _____

   ☞ _____

Learn what truly motivates you, use positive reinforcement, and reward yourself with incentives when you reach your goals.

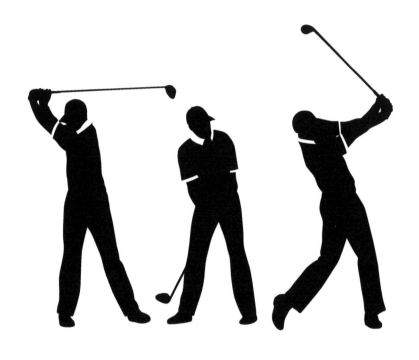

Visualize the Shot

The 13th Hole – Strategy Phase IV:

Visualization and Commitment

Visualization is a creative effort that can be developed and improved over time. You want to move from contemplating change to having a solid picture of change in your mind. You do that by strategically visualizing and then committing to act.

Begin by imagining the outcome you desire, every last detail, to create a lasting image and impression, a vision you can manifest into something real.

The most important aspect of visualization is that your vision needs to be in line with your beliefs. Only then will your mind entertain positive self-talk and thought, reinforcing your vision.

So what does your desired outcome look like, feel like, or even taste like? What do you intend to achieve? Perhaps you want one of the following:

- o To change a belief

- o To upgrade from self-doubt to confidence

- o To achieve a physical feat

- o To lose twenty-five pounds and keep it off

- o To develop a healthful life regimen

- o To feel better and get an A grade on your next physical exam

Next, dig deep to get your originality and creativity in gear, and make this visualization your own. Verbalize it, test-drive it, and pitch it to anyone who will listen. Create a clear, vivid image for your high-concept quest. Your image—your mental vision—will morph and crystallize into something real that you can talk about. It can also act as a switch to allow you to instantly jump into full visualization mode, fully engaged and in pursuit of your intention.

Visualize and commit to a new you

Genuine personal power emanates from living with a sense of awareness: you know yourself well and recognize that you are in control, confident, receptive to positive change, and up for the challenge, any challenge you want to take on.

Take a moment to consider that your body is your physical brand and your mind is the balance of your brand. Branding yourself is the process of visualizing a collection of positive perceptions of yourself. Other people may have different perceptions of your brand, but although you cannot intentionally make people think of your image in a certain manner, you can certainly control the image you put forward for them to interpret. You can also gradually control how you see yourself and feel about yourself.

You, as a brand—really? Yes! Your brand is the promise to yourself—that you are fit, that you are strong, that you are magnificent. If you feel it authentically, others recognize and sense it. Think of branding your whole self—your body, your mind, and your energy.

Now, take that one step further. Think of how the brand you create, the brand that is you, relates to other commercial brands from industry. Think of the ones that best reflect your personal preferences, brand images that you admire. Then start pulling those positive attributes into your awareness. In my case, I wanted to emulate brands that represented determination, resilience, and tenacity.

Now consider the value of your brand. Think of your mind and body as your best and most precious assets. Think of your quality level, perceived value and reputation, as well as your recognition.

Your brand reflects everything that you are—your very essence, what you believe in, value, and exist for. What does that look like? It means how you want people to feel about you and what life role you envision yourself in. Take your mental vision, memorize it, and then carefully build everything else behind it—your confidence, intellect, and integrity. Commit to a new vision of yourself.

In golf, muscle memory refers to the nervous system's ability to memorize or automatically reproduce a motion with which the muscles have become familiar. A solid golf swing is a great example of muscle memory as well as the learned nature of mental and physical success strategies working in tandem. As much as you are mentally visualizing and imagining your swing, you are feeling it and experiencing it. Over time, through repetition, your confidence in your abilities and swing will grow.

Building awareness of your own personal brand is an interesting process of considering how you believe you are perceived as well as how you wish to be.

Visualize realizing your potential

In golf, you work to develop your swing. Over time, you tweak and fine tune and strive for perfection in balance, timing, and tempo. Eventually, you reach a plateau where you will standardize and stabilize a consistent, reliable swing that works for you.

At this plateau, however, the swing may be so ingrained that it can interfere when you try to learn a new and improved swing or technique. You will keep trying to revert to what is comfortable, known, and safe. If that happens, it's crucial to get the old swing completely out of your mind. Don't compare what you are learning to what you've been doing; instead, focus directly on what you are learning, a completely new and fresh start for you and your swing.

I love weight lifting. Aside from enjoying the results, what really resounds with me is the way lifting weights makes me feel. The underlying rule for any weight-lifting program is to stand tall and watch your posture. Strengthening your muscles in turn strengthens your physique, and it doesn't take long before you are walking proudly, with head up and shoulders back. Weight lifting is a way to improve your posture, and you can use it to reshape and transform your body at any age.

Visual and mental aids

You now have some tools—aspirational moxie, TAG lines, and vision. (Have you created your own

TAG line yet?) Pepper this with some eagerness and determination, and your focus and direction will become that much clearer.

Remember our TAG? Here it is again:

T – Thought and Talk: Contemplate and verbally define what you want to achieve.

A – Achieve: What do you hope to achieve or gain? ROI usually means Return On Investment; in this case, it can mean the Rewards Of Imagery. You want your efforts to pay off. It's important to keep this focus in your mind and your vision.

G – Greatness: Success! Rejoice, relive, and do it again!

No Excuses is this book's most important TAG line, but here is another: "When I win in my mind, I win every time."

In 2009, the American Cancer Society launched a major brand revitalization effort that resulted in a wonderfully fresh and warm new TAG line to represent their focus: "The Official Sponsor of Birthdays." Doesn't that make you pause and think? I think it's perfect!

Winners in life visualize their success and look forward to reaping and enjoying the rewards of their accomplishments. They revel in their hard-earned victory, and that reinforces their superior level of self-confidence. Achieving success only serves to rejuvenate their desire and heighten their motivation and commitment. Success fuels their impetus to take excellence to an even higher level, to be the best they can be, and to become even stronger mentally and physically. They become contenders, limitless in their approach to life and ready to take on the world.

At that point they have decided to upgrade from aspiration to expectation, and have begun to visualize an outcome. Something incredibly important has happened. They have committed to the process of change.

The mental visualization drill meets TAG

Want to improve your visualization skills? Create a daily TAG drill.

Begin by imagining every last detail of the outcome you desire to create a lasting image and impression, a vision you can manifest into something real. Perhaps a scenario that adequately reflects your intention and goal will work best. For example, if your intent is to lose twenty-five pounds, contemplate why you want to lose the weight and how you will look and feel when the weight is gone.

Ensure that your vision is in line with your beliefs and be open to positive self-talk and image/intention rehearsals that you can replay in your mind and use to reinforce your vision. Be honest and direct with yourself. You may say you want to lose the weight because you are going to a school reunion and want to look good. If that is the case, after the reunion are you going to gain the weight back? Or have you decided that you really just want to lose the weight and keep it off? If the reunion was the trigger that made you take a good hard look in the mirror and think, *wow, need to do something here*—that's great! Think now. Think me. Think no excuses.

The reunion will come and go, but if you want to get in shape and look better for the reunion, *and* far into the future, it's time for change. Now think of an image or a scenario that lets you envision the new you. Visualize what you will look and feel like once you have lost that weight. Visualize the slimmer, more vibrant you at the reunion, on vacation, dining out, or on the golf course. Billy Crystal's classic TAG line works well here. Think to yourself, "You look marvelous!"

What is your ultimate body dream?

The human body is truly remarkable. Natural beauty and grace of movement—what marvelous gifts we have. When considering the attainment of excellence and your vision of what your ultimate body looks like, keep the following aspects in mind. Visualizing a new, fit, healthier version of yourself starts with developing posture awareness. Walk tall with your head held high and shoulders back. Feel your body and feel in control. The body was never intended to have humps and bumps. The body functions best when it is streamlined, limber, and resilient. Visualize your body as sleek and supple, fine tuned, energetic, and defined.

Do you have a good support system?

Some people can commit and see things through easily. It appears to come naturally for them to finish what they start, but the truth is that they have probably been honing this skill their entire lifetime. Most people, though, achieve more in life when they have a solid support system backing their efforts. This could be in the form of motivational literature, instructional videos, and relevant lectures from influential speakers in conjunction with mentors, coaches, teammates, colleagues, training buddies, and family. The main objective of the support system is to:

- o provide strength and encouragement to keep you going,

- o challenge you to work to your potential,

o reinforce a sense of team spirit where you don't want to let others down, and

o increase your effort by being emotionally tied to wanting a successful outcome and fulfillment.

Support systems guide us to make healthier choices. We have more positive experiences and less chance of depression, and we live longer, build winning habits, stay in control of our lives, and build on our support system with a positive network of people.

Struggle strengthens the human bond and lightens the burden of the human condition

Make a decision to take action and put all your good planning to the test. Ready? For these exercises, I use improved fitness as an example, and I give you a sample response for each. Fill in with your own goals, whether they are on a professional or personal level.

The Lifestyle Prototype

The Visualization and Commitment Phase Summary:

1. Identify projected goal using TAG visualization.

☞ I want overall health improvement, no excuses, visualizing a sleek version of me on the first tee box of my favorite golf course.

☞ _____

☞ _____

2. Identify additional areas for consideration as they relate to your current strategy.

   ☞ Improved core flexibility for power.

   ☞ _____

   ☞ _____

3. Encourage continuing development and commitment to growth and improvement.

   ☞ Practice endurance drills.

   ☞ _____

   ☞ _____

4. Award individuals for their achievements in the success of the overall strategy. Deploy a challenge to encourage others to follow suit.

☛ Achievements and successes shared often create even more focus and direction. Consider the value of standing alone as opposed to standing united. Big quests often need the efforts of a united, committed team.

☛ _____

☛ _____

**_Visualization engages the mind
and encourages the body.
With your visualization intact, commit to act._**

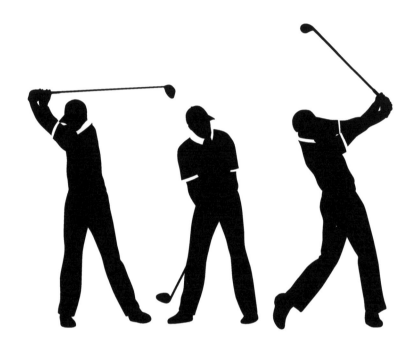

Visualize the Shot

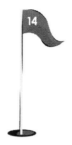

The 14th Hole – **Strategy Phase V:**

Formulate a Curriculum

We visualize in order to develop a solid focus, and at the same time, we develop a keen sense of direction and intention. I typically have four or five active to-do lists with me at any time—a work list, a home list, a fun list, an upcoming events list, and a long-term list. Some are on my iPad and sync to my phone, while others are on paper. For example, at work I like to cross items off my list throughout the day. I like to quickly be able to see at a glance that I am getting things done. At the end of the day I rewrite my list of open items so I'm ready for the next day.

I am big on taking notes. It's how I learned to study. Read, digest, write it out in my own words, summarize in as few words as I can, and commit to memory. Over the years everything important to me—in school, work, or life—has been reprocessed and condensed into a memory, image, catch phrase, or acronym. At that point when I write something out in my own words, I also try to take a new perspective. I challenge myself to use a fresh way of looking at the circumstance or situation. Some of these notes have evolved over the years, flavored by experience and life, and have spawned new life of their own as a thought or quote in one of my books.

This simple task of taking a physical piece of paper and spilling words onto it can be a great beginning if you use it to detail your dreams, your quests, and your priorities. Add to it and upgrade it as you progress. Lists are another form of visual aid.

Be optimistic, be realistic, and be adamant!

The strategy of formulating a curriculum means you need to document your ideas—on paper or electronically—with set objectives, realistic expected outcomes, and a reasonable method of measuring your progress. Consider what you want to benchmark. If fitness is your goal, you can benchmark things like blood pressure, heart rate, cholesterol levels, weight, inches, fat content (body fat percentage), body mass index (BMI), strength, flexibility, club head speed (for the golfers), muscle memory, endurance, and resilience.

What is your fitness motivation and why? Do you want to feel better? Do you want to be muscular and in control of your body? Do you want to be strong, both mentally and physically?

Perhaps it's important for you to be functionally fit, to be able to perform real-life activities, defy the normal process of aging, improve your balance, boost your stamina, and strengthen your core while ridding yourself of annoying aches and pains. Think about developing posture awareness and building your overall strength. Perhaps you want to regenerate and recover from a physical setback or focus on reshaping and remaking your body. Or maybe you are looking to tune up your cardiovascular system and improve your energy levels.

When finalizing your strategy, think improve, enhance, and reduce. The more detailed you are, the better you will be able to define your expected outcome and envision that outcome becoming reality.

What if you could strategically turn back the hands of time?

What if you could look five, ten, even fifteen years younger? Would it be worth the effort for you? I would guess that question just earned a resounding

"Yes!" Is it possible? Yes! You can achieve a more youthful state by simply taking care of your health.

To attain that state, here are some great ideas to begin working into your lifestyle prototype:

1. **Go for a physical exam** – Make having an annual physical a given, including a blood test. A good doctor will listen to your concerns and provide counseling as required. Here is a summary of the information gathered during the physical and subsequent analysis of blood work. Compare your physicals over time to make sure your healthy lifestyle is working for you.

   Vital signs:

   o Blood pressure: Less than 120/80 is a normal blood pressure. High blood pressure or hypertension is defined as 140/90 or higher.

   o Heart rate: Values between 60 and 100 are considered normal, although many healthy people have heart rates slower than 60.

   o Respiration rate: Breathing 16 times per minute is normal, while breathing 20 times or more per minute may suggest heart or lung problems.

o Temperature: Average is 98.6 degrees Fahrenheit (37 degrees Celsius), although healthy people can have a higher or lower resting temperature.

o General appearance: A perceptive doctor can gather a large amount of information about you and your health by watching and talking to you with respect to your memory, your mental prowess and quickness, the appearance of your skin, and your ease of mobility.

Heart exam: By listening to your heart with a stethoscope, your doctor may detect an irregular heartbeat, murmur, or other clues to some form of heart disease.

Lung exam: Also using a stethoscope, your doctor will listen to your breathing. Wheezing, crackling sounds, or limited shallow breathing may be clues to the presence of some form of lung or heart disease.

Head and neck exam: "Open and say *aaaah!*" You know this one. With a full view of your throat and tonsils, your doctor can see the quality of your teeth and gums, which provide information about your overall health. Usually your ears, eyes, nose, sinuses, lymph nodes, thyroid, and carotid arteries will also be examined.

Extra exams: Further examinations may include abdominal, neurological, and dermatological areas and extremities. These may be recommended because of your current health concerns or complaints.

Gender-specific exams may also come into play. For men, a testicular, hernia, penis and/or prostate exam may be warranted. For women, a breast exam, pelvic exam, or pap test may be recommended.

Laboratory tests: Although there is no standard listing of annual physical laboratory tests, here is a sampling of the most commonly administered tests: a complete blood count to measure the concentration of white blood cells, red blood cells, and platelets in the blood, a chemistry panel, a urinalysis, and a lipid panel every five years to check cholesterol levels. For cholesterol, shoot for LDL lower than 130 mg/dl and HDL higher than 40 mg/dl.

For those of you who have more serious concerns, consider having a MRI for early detection of potential life-threatening health issues such as bleeding, tumors, and other abnormalities.

Remember the aspiration-to-expectation concept from the 3rd Hole chapter? Having a physical will provide a beginning point for your fit lifestyle quest, and it will allow you to define the gap you need to fill.

2. **Get your eyes checked** – In addition to evaluating your eyes for glasses and contacts, your optometrist will check your eyes for eye diseases and other problems that could lead to vision loss. During a comprehensive eye exam, your optometrist will evaluate your eyes as an indicator of your overall health. In fact, optometrists often are the first health-care professionals to detect chronic systemic diseases such as high blood pressure and diabetes.

3. **Put yourself first** – Train for you! What do you want?

   o Are you training to excel at a specific sport?

   o Do you want to gain or regain a more youthful appearance?

   o Do you want to reduce your exposure to ill health?

   o Do you want to feel better, mentally and physically?

o Do you want to build your confidence by accomplishing your goals?

4. **Replace worry with wisdom** – People worry about maintaining the brain, eyes, heart, strength, and their stamina. We worry about major causes of premature death such as lung, colon, breast, and prostate cancer, heart disease, and stroke. These provide strong reasons to have your physicals and eye exams on a regular basis. What are your biggest concerns about your lifestyle? Poor nutrition, lack of exercise, feeling constantly tired, weight gain? Do you generally feel like you are too busy to enjoy life? If these sorts of concerns are often present in your mind, *you* could be your own worst enemy.

    Rearrange your priorities and carve out some time for rest and relaxation, and take your health into your own hands. Consider becoming a master detective, chase down possible reasons for your aches and pains and be prepared with knowledge the next time you visit your doctor. Knowledge is everything. No one is more concerned about your health than you are.

5. **Ditch dirty vices** – A few years ago, I attended Bodies, The Exhibition in Montreal, Quebec,

which took visitors through galleries displaying real preserved human bodies. Visitors were provided with an up-close and detailed look inside the skeletal, muscular, reproductive, respiratory, and circulatory systems of the human body.

Human specimens, both male and female, of various sizes and shapes were staged in athletic poses, allowing viewers to imagine the body in motion and engaged in everyday activities. Others were used to illustrate how humans' bad habits cause damage to organs by overeating, lack of exercise, smoking, and alcohol abuse. This exhibition has been shown in various cities and has gained a reputation for altering the way people see themselves and making them more conscious of the need to adopt a healthier lifestyle.

One gallery in particular has stuck in my mind. A body was on display, cut away to show a healthy set of lungs, full, rounded, and bright pink. The next body was cut away in the same manner, instead showing cancerous lungs, misshapen, shriveled and black. It was quite a shocking sight. Next to this display was a large, clear box half filled with what could easily have been several hundred packages of cigarettes. That told the whole story.

6. **Optimize your weight** – Aim to be the right size for your height, sex, age and body type. Keep your waist trim, your body taut, and recover that bounce in your step. Safeguard yourself from disease and take an active role in revitalizing that beautiful body you live in. Don't be a couch crusader. Make lifestyle changes to become more aware of your body and be active each day.

7. **Supplement your eating habits** – It is next to impossible to eat enough of the right foods to get the proper nutrition you need every day, so supplement your diet with a well-balanced multivitamin. Then enhance your nutrition with additional vitamins and nutrients to meet your specific requirements.

8. **Water works** – Commit to drinking eight to ten cups of water each day. What can you expect if you do? Increased strength and endurance. Fewer headaches and less fatigue because you will not be dehydrated. Water regulates your temperature, transports nutrients, and is necessary to build tissue. Water is required for joint lubrication, digestion, circulation, respiration, absorption, and excretion. Water helps your kidneys to efficiently eliminate toxic waste products from your body through urine. Drinking enough water is one of the best things you can do for your health.

Try drinking water before each meal to curb your appetite. Start with half a glass and slowly build up to two glasses.

9. **Get fit with cardio** – A quick blast of cardio gets the blood flowing. Begin your progress with a cardio kick-off to wake up your body and shake off some fat. Take brisk walks, jump on the treadmill, or join some organized cardio classes, either at the gym or at home with a video.

10. **Fuel up with real food** – Start by thinking of food as fuel. If you were a high-performance car, you would likely have a sticker by your fuel tank clearly stating that only premium fuel be used. Moreover, it is highly likely that only the right fuel would be accepted as the wrong fuel nozzle would not fit your tank.

    Well, we are not cars, but our bodies are high performance, and they are spectacular. Given the opportunity to fuel, hydrate, and maintain your body in a manner that will help you to pamper, perfect, and protect it, why would you not? Build a better body by feeding it premium fuel. I'll have more on the right fuel in the next chapter.

11. **Shape up with weights** – Shape and reshape, contour, and define. Train and build the muscle,

strength, and flexibility you need to perform well in the sport or activity of your choice. You can target specific body parts or tone your entire body. Keep your workout cutting edge and interesting. Focus on the muscles that can make your body long and lean and powerful.

12. **Encourage an epic epidermis** – Good health starts on the inside and you will feel it, but it shows on the outside in the texture and overall appearance of your skin. If healthy-looking skin is on your agenda, spend your time and money on your overall fitness, nutrition, and well-being. It will go much further than spending dollars on over-the-counter cure-all creams.

   Note: Be certain to use a good quality sunscreen every day.

13. **Afford time for sleep** – Aim for seven to eight hours of quality sleep every night. I'll admit, I have been known to say, "I'll sleep when I'm dead!" because it seems I'm always busy and running, and there is always so much I want to do that sleep just seems a waste of time. Yet quality sleep is important to your well-being and your ability to deal with the challenges of daily life.

14. **Prosper with a positive mind** – The right attitude is everything, after all. What is the best thing you can bring to an opportunity? Eagerness,

energy, excitement, enthusiasm—it all spells positivity and success.

15. **Live your best lifestyle** – If you want your life to work for you, wherever you have a choice, choose to do the things you like to do best. Develop a lifestyle that is exciting and dynamic, and keep it interesting by constantly growing and learning and changing.

16. **Develop a support team** – Your doctor, your personal trainer, your teammates, your colleagues, your partner or spouse, your friends, your workout partner. Is there someone you love to compete with? Someone who challenges you more than anyone else? Even your favorite opponent can provide support.

17. **Visualize your best body, but manage your current body with respect** – Learn to appreciate how exquisite your body is. Its power, strength, beauty, durability, and capabilities are astounding. Focus on posture, balance, speed, agility, and mobility. Enhance your body's spinal health, flexibility, strength, and muscle tone. Work smart to reduce the risk of injury and work hard to recover from any injuries you do get.

18. **Alter your mind** – The treadmill offers a great time-out luxury for those of us who live hectic lives. You jump on the treadmill, which is great

cardiovascular exercise, so the time-out aspect is easy to justify because you are doing something good for yourself. Within seconds, you are in a groove. You can throw your mind in neutral and let your thoughts wander. Or you can listen to the drone of the treadmill and the slap of your feet—slap, slap, slap. Or you can drown out the slapping with music, or you can pop a DVD into the player and escape into a good movie.

Last year, I bought some DVDs on sale to watch while on the treadmill. One of them was *The Music Within*, the true story of Richard Pimentel, starring Ron Livingston. The caption under the title reads "Anyone can change the world." I think that was why I bought it.

Pimentel's calling in life was helping people with disabilities. He prompted people to alter how they thought about people with disabilities, all disabilities. I was blown away by the story. If you want to see how positive change can impact the world, check this movie out. Another important idea I took away from the movie was not to accept excuses.

Pimentel would not accept being held back because of his disability; moreover, he would not tolerate others trying to hold him back. He changed their minds about prejudging disabilities as being debilitating.

The day I watched that movie, it was a great time-out and a heartfelt blast of inspiration. My favorite quote from the movie was from the very first line, if I recall correctly: "I was born with the umbilical cord wrapped around my neck. I've been pissed off ever since." Well that got me! I was sucked in and paying attention right from the start of the movie, so much so that I completely forgot my time on the treadmill, and the movie was over before I knew it. Brilliant!

Here is a sample of what my lifestyle prototype for this hole can look like. I call it the No Excuses FIT Lifestyle (FIT stands for Focused Intense Training). For these exercises, I use improved fitness as an example, and this time I gave you a full array of sample responses for each. In the section that follows, you can add in your own goals, whether they are on a professional or personal level.

The Lifestyle Prototype

The Formulate a Curriculum Phase Summary:

1. Be credible by clearly documenting your success action plan details—a curriculum for your success.

   ☞ I will create a detailed plan to achieve my overall lifestyle prototype.

☞ My SAP will consist of two key success factors: a healthful diet plan and a physical exercise plan.

☞ The SAP will run for ten weeks.

2. Identify the aspiration, the expectation, and the gap that needs to be filled.

☞ I will lose weight, get in shape, and become healthier overall.

☞ I will begin with a full physical and use key measurable factors from my results such as blood pressure, cholesterol level, weight, and BMI.

☞ I will schedule a follow-up physical to recheck my health status at the end of my ten-week program.

3. Identify the opportunity, the motivation, the incentive, and the desired outcome.

☞ I have every opportunity to complete this program. No excuses.

☞ I am motivated by the sheer fact that I know I will look better and feel better.

☞ My incentive plan will include new golf clothes and a new set of clubs. I am overdue!

☞ My overall desired outcome is twofold: to increase my fitness level and to be toned and tuned up for the upcoming golf season.

4. Detail results as you progress.

☞ I will monitor my progress weekly with mea-surements of expected increases and decreases and my weight.

☞ *I am ready!* Swing thought: FIT = Focused Intense Training.

Okay, your turn!

THE LIFESTYLE PROTOTYPE

The Formulate a Curriculum Phase Summary:

1. Be credible by clearly documenting your suc-cess action plan details—a curriculum for your success.

☞ _____

☞ _____

☞ _____

2. Identify the aspiration, the expectation, and the gap that needs to be filled.

☞ _____

☞ _____

☞ _____

3. Identify the opportunity, the motivation, the incentive, and the desired outcome.

☞ _____

☞ _____

☞ _____

4. Detail results as you progress.

☞ _____

☞ _____

☞ _____

It's not the win that matters so much as recognizing and respecting its value.
True confidence is born of experiencing your hard work and seeing your determination pay off.

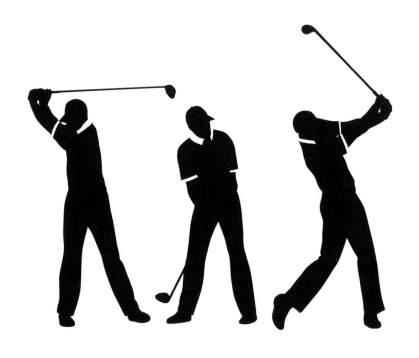

Visualize the Shot

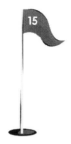

The 15ᵗʰ Hole – Launch Your Success

Action Plan

I'm starting on Monday...yes, really I am!

I have rooted through the pantry, eliminating all the foods that may tempt me to cheat on my new diet. I have my grocery list—a list of healthful, nutritious raw foods. I've checked my stash of vitamins to make certain I have everything I need, and lastly, I've gone to the basement to ensure my treadmill is still there—it is. I have my stack of fitness magazines out on the coffee table and a Victoria's Secret flyer to stick on the fridge that I have been saving for this very moment—my inspiration. Technically, I'm ready.

I must admit that I am very fortunate. I have been blessed with youthful looks, great rock-and-roll hair, and for the longest time, a fast-paced metabolism. Until now, I could eat pretty much anything I wanted and get away with it.

But lately, I've got this jiggle thing happening. I've gained a few pounds, well, maybe fifteen, and I hate it! Time to put the brakes on!

Now let's look at you. Let's take a quick look at preparing to launch your new lifestyle: setting goals, setting the pace, and getting totally psyched.

The mathematics of goal setting

When you find something that works, and it works every time, why would you mess with it? We know that exercise works, and we know that a doctor-approved combination of vitamins and supplements works, so now let's consider what works when it comes to the consumption of food and how to lose fat. The answer? Counting calories. There are many ways to market and remarket this process, many very costly. However, we have a very simple solution here, a mathematical calculation for losing weight that works, and we know that it works every time! There may be some dips and swings from day to day, but you will continue to work toward your right size over the long run. So let's calculate some goals for your daily caloric intake.

Step 1. Calculate your daily caloric needs in order to maintain your weight using a simple formula called the Harris-Benedict principle. Published in 1919 by the Carnegie Institution of Washington, it is based on a study by James Arthur Harris and Francis Gano Benedict to assess your basal metabolic rate (BMR). Your BMR is the amount of energy your body needs to function properly. Approximately 60 percent of the calories we consume daily are used for basic bodily functions such as breathing. Predominant factors that influence your BMR include your weight, height, age, and sex. Use the following formula to calculate your BMR:

For an adult woman:

655 + (4.3 × your weight in pounds) + (4.7 × your height in inches) – (4.7 × your age in years)

Example of a 135 lb. woman, 5'4" tall, aged 40:

655 + (4.3 × 135) + (4.7 × 64") – (4.7 × 40) = 1,348.30 BMR

For an adult man:

66 + (6.3 × your weight in pounds) + (12.9 × your height in inches) – (6.8 × your age in years)

Example of a 171 lb. man, 5'9" tall, aged 40:

66 + (6.3 × 171) + (12.9 × 69") − (6.8 × 40) = 1,761.40 BMR

Step 2. To build activity into your daily caloric needs, do the following calculation:

- o If you are sedentary, take your BMR × 20 percent

- o If you are lightly active, take your BMR × 30 percent

- o If you are moderately active (exercising most days a week), take your BMR × 40 percent

- o If you are very active (exercising intensely on a daily basis or for prolonged periods), take your BMR × 50 percent

- o If you are extremely active (engaging in hard labor or strenuous athletic training), take your BMR × 60 percent

Now add this number to your BMR. Assuming that our examples above are both moderately active the calculation would be as follows:

For an adult woman: 1,348.30 + 539.32 = 1,887.62

For an adult man: 1,761.40 + 704.56 = 2,465.96

This result is the approximate number of calories you can eat every day to maintain your current weight.

Step 3. Next, to lose weight, you have to either create a caloric deficit or exercise at a level higher than the moderate that we used in our calculation in Step 2 to burn calories, or ideally a combination. Note: as you lose weight, recalculate using the formula above to calculate your new BMR. Now let's take a closer look at how to create a caloric deficit.

To lose one pound of fat, you must create a deficit of 3,500 calories by eating less and/or exercising more. Thus, if you create a deficit of 500 calories a day, you will lose one pound a week as a general rule. How does ten pounds in ten weeks sound, or fifty-two pounds a year? Take the weight off in a steady, healthful manner and you will stand a better chance of keeping it off because you are gradually ingraining good habits.

Step 4. Set your target! *GO!*

The simple rule for estimating the ideal weight is as follows:

For women: one hundred pounds for the first five feet and five pounds for each additional inch. Therefore, an average woman at an average height of 5'4" with a medium build should weigh 120 pounds.

For men: one hundred and ten pounds for the first five feet and five pounds for each additional inch. Therefore, an average man at an average height of 5'9" with a medium build should weigh 155 pounds.

The above examples are but one means of calculating your target caloric intake for weight maintenance and weight loss. There are many on the Internet in which you can easily enter a few pieces of data to get an accurate estimate of your body fat and body fat percentage, as well as the calories to be consumed to meet your targeted weight. Some weight-loss apps are available that encourage you to continue to pay attention day after day by sending you a quick alert when you fail to check in.

Pep talk: I used the example above merely as an example from which to springboard. My real intention is to encourage you to stay on track—to not give up as you may have done in the past, but to push on, ingrain your winning habits, and block your excuses.

In praise of exercise

Part of the Success Action Plan launch process involves rekindling your motivation and getting psyched up about what you can achieve. One way is to think back to situations or experiences in which you had a successful outcome. To regain my own desire to commit to exercise, I thought back to my memories and experience of when exercise had had the greatest impact on me. For instance, when I was growing up, my father had back problems. I'm not sure of the cause, but I vividly remember my dad stretched out on his back on the floor in agony. He would go to the chiropractor two or sometimes three times a week, every week. He went to get a "correction," he called it. It always seemed to me that the "correction" didn't work because his prognosis seemed to demand a lifetime of these so-called corrections, with the only alternative being a life spent lying on the floor. Either way, it was not promising.

Then one Christmas a family friend who had suffered a back problem, gave my father a book called *The Back Doctor* by Hamilton Hall, MD (McGraw-Hill, 1980). The book clearly detailed core exercises to build muscle to support one's back. My dad decided not to use the book right away as he seemed to be doing okay at that time. Later, he chalked that up to not being very active for fear he'd throw his back out again. Then one day, after complaining about his back again, he decided it was time to take a read and see whether there was help for him.

"Ten Minutes a Day to Lifetime Relief from Your Aching Back," the cover read. It didn't take long for my dad to prove this to be the truth. Trips to the chiropractor went from three times a week down to two and then one. Then once a month, then once every six months, and then that was it. He was done with the chiropractor. In fact, these straightforward exercises that took only ten minutes a day became an integral part of my father's lifestyle. He soon tripled the exercise reps, doing thirty minutes of core exercises every morning. Then he added a brisk half-hour walk every night after dinner.

I remember visiting my mom and dad in Florida one year. After dinner my dad, then in his early sixties, got up from the table to go for his walk, and mom nudged me out the door with him to keep him company. We laughed and joked around, and I lightly smacked him across the abdomen with the back of my hand. Well, it was as if I had hit my hand on a board. He was all muscle, and I was impressed!

In fact, I had a similar situation. In the spring of 1999, my family moved to a new house on about a half an acre. It had been vacant for two years before we bought it, and as such had a lot of leaves and branches built up around the exterior of the lot in and among the trees. I took on the chore of raking that lawn, planning to plant some flowering shrubs as I went.

I had just finished the front lawn and was starting on the back when I heard a sound I will never forget. It was a high-pitched clicking noise. What was worse than hearing it was that I felt it. The noise had come from me.

From being sticky and overheated from thrashing around in the bush, I went to feeling instantly cold. I felt water trickling from my eyes. I stood still and quiet, afraid to move. Within a few seconds the feeling passed, and I dropped the rake and tried to straighten up. I couldn't move my neck.

I made my way back to the house, and over the next few excruciating hours I worked to relax and straighten up as best I could. I was left with my head tilted slightly to the left and so much pain I thought I would pass out. Subsequent x-rays showed nothing. Doctors said, "Maybe something is just out of place." All I knew for certain was that the pain was very real and it seemed to be building.

I became desperate. Over the next eight-and-a-half months, I visited sports and injury recovery clinics, including seeing several therapeutic masseuses, chiropractors, and even a cranial chiropractor. I was living on pain killers and barely keeping it together. Finally, I decided to look to exercise as my dad had done, but I couldn't do the exercises he was doing—there was too much strain on my neck. I decided to buy a treadmill, thinking that the continual movement would loosen me up and somehow I could work my way through whatever was ailing me.

This first day was tough, but I did it, managing half an hour at a speed of two miles per hour. Afterward I felt broken, but the next morning I felt a little better. On day two, I did half an hour at a speed of three miles per hour, and over the next couple of weeks I worked up to an hour at a speed of four-and-a-half miles an hour. That was as fast as I could walk before breaking into a jog.

By then, the pain was gone and I could move my head freely. Walking on the treadmill would loosen me up and the effects would last a good twenty hours. By the time I stepped on the treadmill for my daily walk, the stiffness and pain had already returned, but each day it improved. This was huge motivation for me to continue, and continue I did— for an entire year I walked five or six times a week for an hour each time, at four-and-a-half miles an hour.

The cottage contingent

My husband and I owned a cottage on an island for just over ten years. We winterized every fall, removing every last scrap of food, and then opened it up again in the spring, restocking for the new season.

Routinely on Friday nights, we would leave our office in the city, drive thirty miles to get home and pick up our daughter, pack, and then jump back in the car for another 160-mile drive to the cottage for the weekend. At the grocery store closest to the cottage, we bought only eggs, brown bread, the best-looking fresh fruit and vegetables, fish or chicken, and meat. The cottage staples consisted of things like olive oil, balsamic vinegar, dried spices, canned tomatoes, pasta, to which we added our fresh food. We purposely bought versatile staples for the season that wouldn't spoil and then supplemented them with only what we needed for the weekend so we wouldn't have a lot of leftovers to lug home.

Gradually, this taught us to combine and mix familiar food in creative new ways. Although we may have repeatedly bought similar foods, we experimented to come up with fresh ideas, new takes on old standards, easy quick healthful food. This becomes important when trying to stick with healthful foods over the long haul and to be able to consistently pass by tempting but unhealthful choices.

Double back and double down

I like this! Double back: turn back the hands of time for a more youthful you. Double down: make a calculated gamble that you hope will maximize the yield of the project. There's much to be gained—big results—if you are willing to do the work.

Have you heard of skin tightening and luminosity? I have heard these terms often with respect to body building. By following an extremely clean diet and working through an intense physical exercise program directed at burning fat and building lean muscle, as you might during the lead-up to a fitness competition, you can both tighten your skin and improve its overall health and appearance.

Now, some would balk at this, and rightfully so. It does seem a tall order to fill. Yet I know first-hand that if you do the work—stick to the diet, take the right vitamins, drink your water, get a good night's sleep, and exercise—you can make a dramatic change in your appearance.

A few years back I bought a book called *Shed 10 Years in 10 Weeks* by Julian Whitaker, MD, and Carol Colman (Simon & Schuster, 1997). I read the book twice and then created a modified personal regimen. The book outlines how to make changes—one a week for ten weeks. It offers a solid overview of nutritional supplements including how to combine them in a safe, nontoxic way.

I was actually already doing most of what was recommended on my own and had been for years, so I didn't roll through the list of changes to be made week by week. No, true to my nature, I was so enticed and excited to get going that I made all the changes I needed to make in the first week and continued well beyond the tenth week. I was also able to recruit my husband and persuade him to join me.

A few months later, I had lost about ten pounds that quite honestly I hadn't thought I needed to lose. But I had, and I felt terrific. As a matter of course, my next physical was coming up. The results? Outstanding—so much so that my doctor asked what I was doing. Other people also asked both my husband and I what we were doing differently. The changes were obvious. There was a big difference in the new growth of my fingernails and in the color and texture of my new growth of hair. The physical change before and after was astounding.

I continued to buy this book again and again. I always seemed to end up telling someone about it and then giving them my copy and having to buy it again. Over the years, I have continued to learn what works and what doesn't, and I've perfected my own lifestyle program—the No Excuses Success Action Plan, which has evolved from thirty years of tweaking and perfecting.

Little lifestyle changes can add up to big results!

Here is the thing about creating a lifestyle. It's the little things that count and little things that add up over time. You make subtle changes that may be of little or no consequence on their own, but gradually those mini efforts take on a life of their own. Here are some examples:

o Lose the office chair, sit on a Swiss ball, and burn more calories from nine to five.

o Lose the juice and eat fresh whole fruit. One medium orange contains sixty-two calories, twelve grams of sugar, and three grams of fiber, while an eight-ounce glass of orange juice from concentrate contains 110 calories, twenty-four grams of sugar, and little to no fiber. Your body has to work to digest the orange, which results in burning calories, but the processed orange juice is ready energy, which, if you don't use it, it is likely to be stored as fat.

o When you go anywhere with a crowded parking area, park away from the entrance. Save your car from door chips, and burn some calories on your walk.

o Plan to eat what you crave in moderation as a reward for losing weight instead of eating something unplanned just because it's in front of you.

o   Do thirty crunches, pushups, or jumping jacks three times a day.

o   Check your posture and stretch tall every time you are in front of a mirror.

o   Set your electric toothbrush to a three-minute setting. While you brush your teeth, do leg lifts, alternating the style on alternate days. On day one, bend and lift your knees to the front, and on day two, lift your legs straight to the side.

o   Eliminate the bad foods from your diet, the foods that have no chance of ever registering on the healthy scale. No nutritional value, too many calories, too much sugar or fat—not going to happen! It's not worth the temptation. You have worked too hard!

Counteract the cravings with these healthful tips:

The following is a list of healthful tips to combat the cravings.

o   Instead of eating ice cream, opt for frozen bananas or strawberries.

o Instead of popsicles, frozen red grapes make a refreshing treat.

o Fresh fruits like strawberries, pineapple, or orange sections are a wonderful treat when half dipped in semi-sweet dark chocolate.

o Say no to high-cal chips and chomp on oven-roasted pumpkin or squash seeds or toasted chickpeas. Try kale chips. You simply de-stem and wash the kale leaves, rub them in olive oil, place them on a foil-covered baking sheet, and bake them until crisp. Sea salt optional.

o Air popped popcorn is magnificent. Heat some coconut oil. Sprinkle with black or cayenne pepper, mixing slightly, and then let sit for a few minutes so the pepper flavor infuses the oil. Then add the popcorn ker-nels and pop.

o For pasta dishes, aside from using the fail-safe spaghetti squash, you can substitute parboiled julienned zucchini and carrots. For lasagna, use baby spinach leaves as a base and layer pasta on top, followed by the sauce, using only half of the regular amount of pasta called for.

o If you can't break away from the odd dollop of butter, in a blender combine equal amounts of slightly softened unsalted butter and cold-pressed extra-virgin olive oil, and you'll have a healthful, spreadable butter alternative.

o In place of lasagna noodles, use eggplant or zucchini strips lightly sautéed in olive oil.

o Use butter lettuce (also known as Boston or Bibb lettuce) for wraps instead of bread or pitas.

o Instead of eating crackers, peel a thick broccoli stalk, then slice it into wafer thin rounds. Carrots also work well.

o Greek-style plain yogurt with a spritz of lime is a great substitution for sour cream.

o Mashed or blended avocado works well in place of mayonnaise.

o And here is one of my favorites. Instead of consuming high calorie juices or sodas, steep some flavored tea and chill in a large jug. Then add some sliced citrus fruits for additional flavor and color and serve over ice.

See the next chapter for more of my healthy food ideas and recipes.

Keep thinking—little changes, big results

So you've made up your mind. You recognize the importance and value of exercise, hydrating, vitamins and supplements, controlling your caloric intake, and eating healthfully, and you have the desire to be the right size. Just remember—please check with your doctor before significantly changing your diet or starting a new exercise plan. Not only will it ease your mind to know that you are making good choices, but he or she may have literature or information to specifically target your individual needs.

You may have heard the phrase, "live today as if there's no tomorrow." Great for the attitude, not so great for the body! How about this instead:

Live today as if there will be many tomorrows!

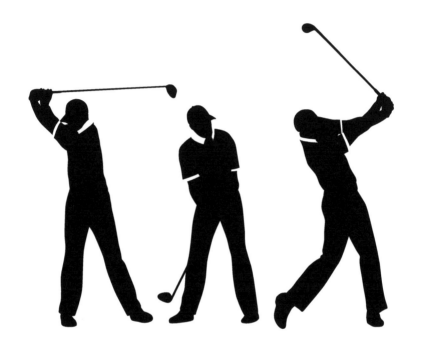

Visualize the Shot

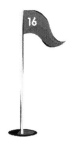

The 16th Hole – The No Excuses FIT Lifestyle

I was a skinny kid growing up. I had long legs and I could run fast, which for me meant I played a lot of sports. In public school, I played soccer. In middle school, I played volleyball. In high school, I ran track. In college, I panicked, thinking that I was much too skinny, and I began lifting weights. In my early twenties I played flag football—not well, mind you—but I could catch the ball and I could run.

In 1996, I decided to get serious about getting in shape. I joined a fitness gym, got a trainer, and committed to working out six hours a week for a full year. I did an hour of cardio followed by an hour of weights three times a week. I stuck it out for the year and managed to get my body fat percentage down to 8 percent.

Life went on, and I continued to be relatively active until 1999, when, as I mentioned on the fifteenth hole, I wrenched my neck one day while raking our yard. It was a strange fluke of an accident that led me to literally walk away my pain with a full year on the treadmill. In 2002, once again I decided it was time to get in shape and committed a year to Pilates, fifty minutes five times a week.

In 2005, I took up golf. Since then, I walk the course whenever possible, and I now exercise in a different way. I want a flexible core and increased strength so I use fitness-to-function training, meaning I exercise specifically to be able to improve at my sport of choice.

Oh, and as for the skinny kid problem, it's long gone!

What does appropriate weight mean?

It's really not about the weight, is it? It is about your fitness level. You may fit nicely into your clothes and generally look good, and maybe you're thinking that you don't need to bother with this lifestyle prototype because you look okay. But just because you are thin, or weight appropriate, does not mean you are in good health.

Good health and wellness build from the inside out. They don't just happen; they take hard work and time. But it is worth it. Please don't make excuses for not taking my challenge because you feel you are weight appropriate. It is important for everyone to take responsibility for the quality of their lives and the condition of their health.

I'll take a slim, toned physique,
some good all-around health,
some strength and flexibility,
and, oh yes, some endurance.
And for dessert, let me see...okay,
I'll take a youthful appearance topped
with some kick-ass confidence.
That's all, thank you!
If only it were that easy!

An important reason for my ability to lose weight quickly is that I manage and control my food cravings. I do this by using the food tips at the end of the previous chapter and also by being focused on results. I think of food as fuel, and I build a great cardio workout plan that's fun and versatile to burn calories. Then, knowing that seeing quick results will keep my focus at an optimal level, I supplement my regimen with a strict, healthful, calorie-reduced diet. I want to feel full and burn the excess fat off.

When I regard food as fuel, I am much less tempted by unhealthful foods. I am big on getting results, especially up front, as it instills a sense of accomplishment for me. I tell myself I am going to build my mind and body into the most efficient machine possible—look at what I have achieved already!

With respect to my diet, I eat clean. In my twentieth year, I developed an extreme allergy to food additives. Although I always carry antihistamines and adrenalin needles, I choose to avoid foods that may contain the mystery chemical that sends me running frantically to emergency. Even with these precautions, this has happened too many times for my liking. Because the allergy testing I have done over the years has failed to specifically identify which additives I should avoid with accuracy, I avoid as many as possible.

Think of food as fuel for your mind and body

Healthful, nutritional food is the fuel for your mind and body. It is the foundation of performance in every area of leading an exciting, active, successful life. Natural foods in their raw state will make you feel lighter, stronger, and more vibrant. You can eat to release toxins naturally and lose weight, if needed. You can also improve your skin quality and health through diet so you look more youthful—the outward indication of inner rejuvenation. You can literally feed your brain in order to help you function and think better.

A good diet has restorative powers and will make you feel good. You can increase your stamina, counter the effects of aging, maintain a healthful weight, and increase your energy. A healthful diet will focus on losing fat rather than a combination of muscle, water, and fat. Your goal is to lose the fat and keep the muscle. Muscle requires more calories to maintain it, but it also means that muscle has more calorie-burning power, so there's a definite benefit to building and retaining lean muscle.

My No Excuses FIT (Focused Intense Training) diet philosophy is my lifestyle now. It has evolved over the last thirty years. It is straightforward and simple, especially when you consider the reasons behind it. A healthful lifestyle evolves when you find the right combination of healthful eating habits and activity level that you can live with long term. Here are the basics:

The No Excuses FIT Lifestyle – Focused Intense Training

Here is a quick breakdown of the components of a healthful diet:

> ☞ 50 percent of your diet should consist of quality proteins, lean red meat, skinless chicken and turkey, fish, shellfish, eggs/egg whites (one yolk for every five egg whites),

low or nonfat dairy products, and beans, nuts and seeds.

~ 30 to 35 percent of your diet should consist of a combination of complex carbohydrates. Fibrous carbs are a dieter's dream. Fiber cannot be digested, and the body burns a lot of energy or calories in the attempt. Complex fibrous carbohydrates include vegetables such as asparagus, broccoli, Brussels sprouts, cabbage, carrots, cauliflower, celery, collard greens, cucumber, green beans, kale, lettuce, mushrooms, okra, peas, peppers (red, yellow, or green), salads, spinach, squash, tomatoes, turnip, and zucchini. Fruits include apples, bananas, berries, cantaloupe, grapefruit, grapes, nectarines, oranges, peaches, pears, and plums. Complex starchy carbohydrates include 100 percent whole-grain dry cereals, wheat or whole-grain pasta, wheat bread and whole-grain products, beans, lentils, legumes, brown rice, oatmeal, cream of rice, cream of rye, cream of wheat, potatoes (red or white), yams, and sweet potatoes.

~ 15 to 20 percent of your diet should include healthful fats such as fish oils, nuts and seeds, natural peanut butter, olives, and vegetable oils like canola, flaxseed, and olive oil.

↜ Take a daily multi-vitamin.

↜ Eat six or more small meals a day.

↜ Drink six to eight glasses of water a day.

↜ Say no to fruit juices, all forms of processed foods, and growth hormones.

↜ Cut out sugar and salt.

In addition to a healthful diet:

↜ Do cardiovascular exercise for fat loss at least three times a week.

↜ Lift weights to tone and build muscle and bone density at least three times a week.

Sustenance! Your health is always the best prescription

I refer to food as fuel for two distinct reasons. First, it shifts how I think and feel about food. The function of food is to supply energy and nutrients to the body thus making eating for taste and gratification secondary. That doesn't mean you shouldn't enjoy the taste of what you eat, but an understanding of what you should eat will lead you to make better choices. Second, when I eat mindfully and healthily, I can tell when my diet is working properly for me. Shortly after I have ingested healthful food, my core temperature rises. I can feel my metabolism kicking in, converting the food into clean fuel.

Let's look more closely at the main food-for-fuel groups. Food consists of three macronutrients:

Protein – Your body, after water, is mostly made of protein. You require protein every day to effectively perform thousands of functions in the body. It does this with different combinations of amino acids, which are the building blocks of protein. Your body uses protein to repair tissue, build muscle, and carry vitamins and hormones throughout the body through the bloodstream.

Carbohydrates – Carbohydrates are the preferred form of fuel for the body's energy needs. Simple or sugary carbs have their place, but for the most part you should eat complex or slow-burning carbs. An important point about carbs and where the average person makes a mistake is that after you supply your immediate energy needs, any excess carbs will be stored as fat. Complex fibrous carbs are dietary superheroes because they are rich sources of vitamins, minerals, phytochemicals, and other nutrients. And they are full of fiber, the indigestible portion of plant material, which means that much of the food passes directly through your system without being absorbed. Fiber is a great colon cleanser and is essential for maintaining a healthy digestive system. But the best thing about fibrous carbohydrates is that they are very low in calories, and it is virtually impossible to overeat on green vegetables. In fact, some vegetables are so low in calories they contain fewer calories than your body requires to process them. For example, a raw celery stick contains approximately five calories, but the body will burn about ten calories just breaking down, assimilating, and eliminating the celery stick, therefore creating a calorie deficit. So eat as many leafy green vegetables as you possibly can.

Grains, seeds, beans and legumes – Reach for the foods that when ready to eat are as close as possible to their original, raw, unprocessed state. As much as this applies to all foods, it is extremely important when selecting grains, seeds, beans and legumes for your diet. And the winners are: Grains – oatmeal, seeds – quinoa and bulgur, beans and legumes – soy beans, red beans, kidney beans, pinto beans and garbanzo beans.

Tip: Mixed beans marinated in a light Italian dressing are great served on a bed of mixed greens.

Fats – There are healthy fats such as monounsaturated fats, polyunsaturated fats and plant sterols. They transfer some vitamins through your bloodstream and help your body store energy. A quick rule of thumb to recognize healthy fats is that they are usually liquid.

Monounsaturated fats: Canola, olive and peanut oils are the healthiest fats you can eat. They lower LDL (bad cholesterol) and raise HDL (good cholesterol) in the blood which aids in lowering the risk of heart disease.

Polyunsaturated fats: Corn, flaxseed, safflower, soybean and sunflower oils, as well as the oils in fatty fish such as salmon are essential for good health. They are rich in omega-3 and omega-6 fatty acids and aid in lowering total cholesterol, both LDL and HDL.

Plant sterols: Nuts, seeds, cereals and legumes contain substances called plant sterols. They aid in slowing the absorption of dietary cholesterol and can lower LDL and total cholesterol in the blood.

There are also harmful fats such as saturated fats, trans fats, and cholesterol. A quick rule of thumb to recognize harmful fats, they are usually solid or semisolid at room temperature turning to liquid when heated.

Saturated fats: These fats are predominant in meat, dark-meat poultry and poultry skin, butter, full fat dairy, coconut oil, and palm oil. They increase total blood cholesterol and LDL.

Trans fats: Hydrogenated oils as found in solid stick margarine and shortening raise total blood cholesterol and LDL levels.

Cholesterol: Egg yolk, liver, shellfish, and full fat dairy are high in cholesterol which can raise blood cholesterol, although interestingly it doesn't in all people.

Unfortunately, most of us eat far too much of the bad fats that over time can increase your risk for heart disease and various forms of cancer, yet proper food choices and moderation can take care of this problem. Aim to keep your daily cholesterol intake less than 300 milligrams.

By reducing your salt, sugar, and bad fats, and by managing your total calorie consumption, you can quickly take control of the food portion of the healthful lifestyle equation.

Managing the macronutrients

With this balance in mind, you stack your carb intake a little higher on your weight-training days to provide enough energy. Then cut back on your carb intake on cardio days, as you'll lose fat faster if you work out on an empty stomach. Staggering your carb intake from high to low day to day in conjunction with your change from cardio to weights will also work in your favor to burn calories.

Familiarize yourself with the glycemic index or GI, which is a measure of a food's ability to elevate blood sugar, and the glycemic load, which is the glycemic index of a food multiplied by its carbohydrate content in grams, which tells you the carbohydrate level in a food.

For years, I've used the plan I've outlined, and it can work for you too. You will determine your portion sizes based on the calorie content of each food choice and your daily personal needs. Fibrous carbs are a good choice because the body does not digest them; you can eat plenty of this type of food and not have to worry about fat storage.

As well, you can enjoy low or no fat, low or no sugar dessert-type foods to keep a plan like this from being too bland. You can also use low or no sodium seasoning to add flavor to meats.

Jalapeno, habanero, and cayenne peppers are also great for adding flavor. Drink coffee and green tea in moderation.

Note: If you don't want the caffeine, drink decaffeinated coffee or tea, but don't shy away from these nearly calorie-free drinks. They are a great source of antioxidants.

Eat foods to promote health and prevent disease

Let's now take an even closer look. I chose the foods listed in this book based on their fat-burning characteristics in combination with offering balanced nutrition, a high antioxidant value, low glycemic index, and conservative calorie level. They are my staples.

The caloric and fiber food values listed below were adapted from: U.S. Department of Agriculture, Agricultural Research Service. 2002. USDA Nutritive Value of Foods, Home and Garden Bulletin Number 72. Source: http://www.ars.usda.gov/Services/docs.htm?docid=6282

Try a One Day Metabo Blast

Looking to boost your willpower and tip the scale in your favor? Take a low-cal fruit and veggie break once every couple of weeks. Pick a few low-cal fruits and vegetables, cut them up into bite-sized pieces, organize them into small packets, and eat one packet every half hour throughout the day with water or decaffeinated coffee or tea.

Exercising your willpower in this manner has twice the impact. You'll prove to yourself that you can get through a twenty-four-hour period eating exceptionally well, and you'll see results in improving your eating habits that much more quickly. It's a win-win!

Complex Fibrous Carbs: Each of the following raw fruits and vegetables has around twenty to forty calories per the portion size listed below. Eat them raw or steamed on the half-hour—but no dip or dressing allowed. Mix them up and have fun with this. Challenge your friends and colleagues to join you.

Fruits	Measure	Calories	Fiber(g)	GI
Apples	¼ fruit	20	0.9	39
Berries	¼ cup	20	1.0	50
Cantaloupe	½ cup	28	0.7	65
Grapefruit	½ fruit	39	1.3	25
Grapes, seedless, green	10 grapes	36	1.6	46
Nectarines	½ fruit	33	1.1	42
Oranges	½ fruit	31	1.5	42
Peaches	½ fruit	21	1.0	42
Pears	¼ fruit	24	1.0	38
Plums	1 fruit	36	1.0	39

Vegetables	Measure	Calories	Fiber(g)	GI
Asparagus	5 spears	18	1.3	14
Beans, green	½ cup	22	2.0	15
Broccoli	1 cup	25	2.6	10
Brussels Sprouts	⅓ cup	20	1.4	16
Cabbage	1 cup	18	1.6	10
Carrots	⅓ cup	24	1.7	49
Cauliflower	1 cup	25	2.5	15
Celery	3 stalks	18	2.1	15
Collard greens	½ cup	25	2.7	15
Cucumber	1 ½ cups	21	1.2	15
Kale	½ cup	18	1.3	15
Lettuce	2 ½ cups	18	2.0	10
Mushrooms	1 cup	18	0.8	10
Okra	½ cup	26	2.0	15
Peas, sugar snap	½ cup	18	1.0	15
Peppers	1 medium	18	0.7	15
Salad, mixed greens	2 ½ cups	20	2.0	10
Spinach	3 cups	21	2.4	15
Squash	1 cup	23	2.1	15
Tomatoes	1 medium	26	1.4	15
Turnip	¾ cup	25	2.3	72
Zucchini	1 cup	23	2.1	15

This sort of a one-day blast works great for me because I am often so busy that I don't have a lot of time for preparation. I like quick, clean, healthful food that's ready in a snap. Besides this One Day Metabo Blast, I have come up with a flexible daily menu that requires minimal prep time, can be easily altered to include the best-looking produce of the day, and gives you the opportunity to have as much variety as you require.

In my No Excuses FIT food planner, a day's worth of six meals can be quickly orchestrated. For fish, please check calories based on the actual fish used. As this is a guide, adjust as required to suit your daily caloric needs as calculated in the last chapter.

Meal One
breakfast: Choose one of the following:

> 1 package oatmeal or cream of wheat (120 calories)
> 6 egg whites, scrambled or fried in a healthful oil (120 calories)
> 1 scoop of low-calorie protein powder (120 calories)
>
> Plus two or three of the following:
> ½ large grapefruit or ½ apple (40 calories)
> 10 seedless grapes (35 calories)
> 1 nectarine or 1 orange (65 calories)
> 1 peach or 1 plum (40 calories)
> ½ banana or ½ pear (50 calories)
> ½ cup raspberries, strawberries, or watermelon (25–35 calories)

Meal Two
breakfast/lunch: Choose one of the following:

½ package oatmeal or cream
of wheat (60 calories)
4 egg whites, scrambled or fried
in a healthful oil (80 calories)
⅔ scoop of low-calorie protein
powder (80 calories)

Plus two or three of the following:
½ large grapefruit or ½ apple
(40 calories)
10 seedless grapes (35 calories)
1 nectarine or 1 orange (65
calories)
1 peach or 1 plum (40 calories)
½ banana or ½ pear (50 calories)
½ cup raspberries, strawberries,
or watermelon (25–35 calories)

Meal 3
afternoon meal: Choose one of the following:

26 whole almonds, oil roasted
cashews or peanuts (165 calories)
1 tbsp. peanut butter and 1 slice
whole wheat or whole grain
bread (165 calories)
3 oz. poultry, light meat, boneless
and skinless (170 calories)

3 oz. fish (100 calories
approximately, varies by type)

Plus two or three of the following:
½ cup yam, peeled, ½ white
potato, peeled, or ⅓ cup
cooked brown rice (75 calories)
1 cup broccoli or 1 cup
cauliflower (25 calories)
¼ cup carrot, 1½ cups cucumber,
1 medium sized pepper, or ½ cup
tomato (20 calories)
½ cup green beans, ⅓ cup
onion, 1 cup mushrooms, or
3 cups spinach (20-25 calories)
2 cups mixed greens, 6 tbsp.
salsa, or 5 asparagus spears
(20–25 calories)

Meal 4
afternoon meal: Choose one of the following:

1 cup high fiber, low sugar (less
than 5 grams) cereal and 1 cup
skim milk (196 calories)
20 pecan halves (196 calories)
4 oz. lean ground beef, 5% fat
(285 calories)

Plus two or three of the following:

½ cup yam, peeled, ½ white potato, peeled, or ⅓ cup cooked brown rice (75 calories)
1 cup broccoli or 1 cup cauliflower (25 calories)
¼ cup carrot, 1½ cups cucumber, 1 medium sized pepper, or ½ cup tomato (20 calories)
½ cup green beans, ⅓ cup onion, 1 cup mushrooms, or 3 cups spinach (20-25 calories)
2 cups mixed greens, 6 tbsp. salsa, or 5 asparagus spears (20–25 calories)

Meal 5
evening meal: Choose one of the following:

1 cup cottage cheese, uncreamed (125 calories)
1 cup soy milk (81 calories)
48 pistachio nuts (161 calories)
3 oz. poultry, light meat, boneless and skinless (170 calories)
3 oz. fish (100 calories approximately, varies by type)

Plus two or three of the following:
½ cup yam, peeled, ½ white potato, peeled, or ⅓ cup cooked brown rice (75 calories)

1 cup broccoli or 1 cup
cauliflower (25 calories)
¼ cup carrot, 1½ cups
cucumber, 1 medium sized
pepper, or ½ cup tomato
(20 calories)
½ cup green beans, ⅓ cup
onion, 1 cup mushrooms, or 3
cups spinach (20-25 calories)
2 cups mixed greens, 6 tbsp.
salsa, or 5 asparagus spears
(20–25 calories)

Meal 6
evening meal: Choose one of the following:

½ cup buttermilk (232 calories)
Tofu, soft, (2 ½ x 2 ¾ x 1) fried in
Memmi noodle soup base and
olive oil (133 calories)
3 oz. poultry, light meat, boneless
and skinless (170 calories)
3 oz. fish (100 calories
approximately, varies by type)

Plus salad made of lettuce,
tomato, and cucumber
(25 calories)
1 tsp. low calorie salad dressing
(10 calories)

Following are some of my go-to recipes that you can easily incorporate into your meal planning:

The Clean Protein Salad

3 oz. tuna, canned, packed in water (70 calories)
1 tsp. olive oil (60 calories)
1 tsp. capers (1 calorie)
1 tbsp. diced red onion (10 calories)
1 hard-boiled egg (80 calories)
2 cups chopped or torn lettuce (14 calories)
1 tsp. mustard (5 calories)

Mix and serve or fold into your favorite leafy green and serve like a taco.

Yield: 2½ cups at 240 calories or two 1¼-cup servings at 120 calories each.

Easy Cucumber Salad

2 cups chopped cucumber (28 calories)
1 cup grape tomatoes cut into halves (60 calories)
2 oz. low-fat part-skimmed-milk mozzarella cheese, cubed (20 calories)
¼ cup diced fresh basil (1 calorie)
1 tsp. olive oil (60 calories)
1 tbsp. balsamic vinegar (5 calories)
Pepper to taste

Mix and serve.

Yield: 3 cups at 174 calories or three 1-cup servings at 58 calories.

Citrus Chicken Salad

¼ cup plain nonfat yogurt (20 calories)
1 tsp. orange or lemon juice (10 calories)
1 8" celery stalk (6 calories)
1 pound boneless skinless chicken, diced and sautéed in olive oil (600 calories)
1 medium tart green apple, diced (80 calories)
½ cup seedless grapes, halved (60 calories)
¼ cup toasted raw almonds (138 calories)

Mix and serve or cut calories in half by serving ½ cup of the citrus chicken salad on a bed of healthful greens.

Yield: 5 cups at 914 calories or five 1-cup servings at 183 calories each.

The Modest Caprese Salad

½ cup low-fat cottage cheese (40 calories)
¼ cup diced fresh basil (1 calorie)
2–3 thick slices of red vine tomatoes (35 calories)
2 tbsp. balsamic vinegar (10 calories)

Mix and serve.

Yield: One 1-cup serving at 86 calories.

The No-Excuses Soup

6 cups low-fat, low-sodium chicken or beef broth
(60 calories)
1 28-oz. can diced tomatoes with juice (160 calories)
2 tbsp. tomato paste (30 calories)
4 cups cabbage, chopped (72 calories)
1 cup onion, chopped (61 calories)
1 cup carrots, sliced (70 calories)
1 cup green beans (44 calories)
1 cup zucchini, chopped (23 calories)
¼ cup fresh basil, diced (1 calorie)
¼ cup fresh oregano, diced (1 calorie)
¼ cup fresh garlic, diced (20 calories)
Pepper to taste

Sauté onions, garlic, and carrots for fifteen
minutes in large pot. Add all other ingredients
and simmer for one hour.

Yield: 12 cups at 542 calories or twelve 1-cup
servings at 45 calories.

Can you think of food as fuel and still have fun with it? Think outside the kitchen!

Try to think of food as a creative venture, a
delectable source of sensory pleasure, and a
great way to gain some control over your health

and weight while enjoying some sumptuous sustenance.

I love the winter holiday season, all the treasures it brings, getting together with family, making time to rekindle friendship, and taking the opportunity to reflect on the passing of another year. A couple of years ago, it seemed as though everyone we knew was having a Christmas party, a pre-New Year's party, or a New Year's Party. There were even after parties.

One New Year's Eve party, however, stands out in my mind. We had an intimate dinner with close friends just outside of town. Their house sat high on a hill overlooking a valley. Secluded and surrounded by tall, snow-laden trees, it was a perfect backdrop for a fabulous night.

Their house contained a "Muskoka" room. Muskoka is "cottage country" in Ontario, one of the province's most visited areas, especially in the summer. Known for its beautiful rugged scenery and clean air, it is Ontarians' destination of choice to escape urban life, and builders have tried to incorporate that sense of vacation and retreat into the design of their new homes.

A Muskoka room is attached to the house but has no inner doors—one enters by going outside and then back in through an outside door. It's much like having your cottage or cabin a few steps away from your house—convenient, but you actually feel as if you are away somewhere else. In my friends' house, the room was about sixteen by thirty feet, and when you looked out through the floor-to-ceiling windows, you could feel the full wonder of winter with the moonlight breaking through the falling snow. Inside the room, the fire set the tone, the hiss and crackle of the burning wood and slight scent of stale smoke spelling instant relaxation.

So, there we were, on New Year's Eve, enjoying wine by the fire, when our friends brought in a raclette to cook some appetizers. I had seen a variation of the raclette in Banff years before. Back then, I tried to buy one but couldn't find them anywhere, but now they seem to be everywhere. A raclette is a form of compact indoor grill, like a fondue alternative, but it heats up in seconds and has no messy oil to contend with.

Random appetizers on a raclette

This was certainly thinking outside the kitchen. We had scallops, shrimp, cheeses, and assorted colorful julienned vegetables accompanied by bottles of fine wine. It was magnificent.

Of course, knowing that I was about to start my No Excuses fitness regimen, I was quickly captivated with the raclette. After New Year's, I headed out to buy one. A few days later, my husband and I cooked an exquisite raclette meal of tuna, calamari, and vegetables—all very healthful. A couple of days later, we had friends come to visit from the city, and they cooked a feast on the raclette. Again, very healthful!

Even when counting calories, you can throw together a healthful, low-cal meal in minutes. Minimal prep time, minimal mess, and just a little inspiration is all it takes.

Invoke some creative cookery and out-chef yourself

Possibly the toughest part of eating well as part of a healthy lifestyle is dealing with the social aspect of it. How can you eat healthful meals without falling into temptation while dining out? How can you still eat with your family without cooking separate meals? Seriously, who has time to prepare a separate dinner every night for themselves when the rest of the family has to be fed regular meals?

The solution? One of my favorite books is called *The 150 Healthiest 15-Minute Recipes on Earth* (Jonny Bowden and Jeanette Bessinger, Fair Winds Press, 2010), one hundred and fifty nutritious, fast, and tasty meals to choose from, lots of pictures, and calorie and macronutrient breakdowns by serving. And if one of the servings has too many calories for your program, cut the serving size down and serve it on a bed of greens. Improvise!

Improving your health and wellness is something you can do for you. You may start out striving to feel better and stronger, but don't discount the fact that you are going to look better too. A healthful diet promotes youthfulness and radiance. Perhaps you have some favorite recipes that you can overhaul?

Getting results is always the goal!

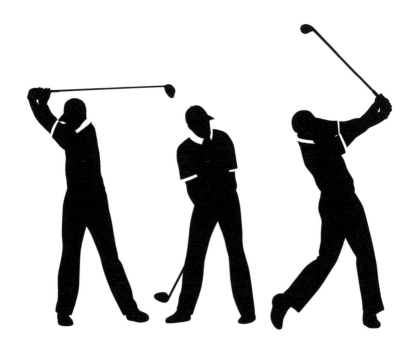

Visualize the Shot

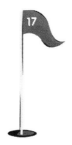

The 17th Hole – **Exercise Your Options**

Golf requires a surprising amount of strength and stamina. You need to attack the hole, strike with precision to make accurate contact with the ball, and go for the shot aggressively. It is always better to be just past your target than to fall short of it.

Many recreational golfers adopt a "swing lightly" mentality, meaning they do not put a lot of *oomph* into the ball. They do so because they have found that they can hit the ball squarely more frequently if they do not swing through with as much club head speed. Therefore, they simply lose the will to be aggressive and progressive in honing their physical skills. They lose their edge, choosing to play it safe rather than pushing past their barriers to become a better golfer.

Rationalizing exercise—it's all positive!

This brings us to the exercise portion of the lifestyle prototype quest, in which, having checked our excuses at the door, we have committed to a spectacular and dramatic journey into the land of the fit.

Back on the fifteenth hole, we looked at how to lose one pound by creating a caloric deficit. To recap: to lose one pound of fat, you must create a deficit of 3,500 calories by eating less and/or exercising more. Thus, if you create a deficit of 500 calories a day, you will lose one pound a week as a general rule.

We have discussed the No Excuses FIT Lifestyle, and you may have a similar healthful plan that has worked for you in the past that you want to resurrect. It's all good, as long as you are staying within your optimal daily caloric intake levels.

The next plan is the exercise plan. Why? Because it is much better to burn fat off than to diet it off. With exercise combined with proper nutrition, you can burn excess body fat, feed your muscles, and elevate your metabolism. Diet without exercise may lead to drastic calorie slashing, which lowers your metabolic rate. This causes your body to invoke the starvation response and begin to store fat, decreasing lean body mass and resulting in muscle atrophy.

Eating six or more small meals a day boosts your metabolism, as does cardio exercise. Cardio refers to any cardiovascular activity that is rhythmical in nature, involves large muscle groups, and can be sustained for long periods of time. For example, if you take a cart when golfing, that would be called a recreational sport. But if you walk the course, carry your clubs, and don't have to wait behind players in front of you, golf turns into a form of aerobic exercise—and a good one, considering the three-and-a-half to four hours it takes to play one round.

A few years ago, I heard about a kind of golf race that was played in teams of four (it was a fundraiser). Each player had a choice of three clubs to play with, which they were to carry in a satchel similar to one you might use to carry a bow and arrow. The players were to hit the ball off the first tee in turn and then run to it, take their next shot, and carry on. Each player was timed independently from the first hole to the ninth, given a short break, and then timed from the tenth hole to the eighteenth. At the end of the round, the four team members' times and golf scores were added together to find the winners. Of course, in a race like this, it would help to be a good golfer, a good runner, and in good health overall. But anyone who golfs for exercise and pleasure can do it. It would also trim the time it takes to play a round of golf. Special arrangements would have to be made to organize such a game, but it would certainly make for a fun and challenging workout.

Cardio is one of the most important things you can do for your body—to lose weight, to build muscle, and to improve your overall health. Decreased blood pressure, decreased blood cholesterol, lowered resting heart rate, and increased aerobic capacity can be achieved in as little as twelve to twenty minutes of daily cardiovascular activity. Choices abound for cardio exercise—a good thing, because variety is important when working to create a healthful lifestyle. You can do almost anything that gets your heart rate into your target heart-rate zone. (A target zone is a heart-rate range that guides your workout by keeping your intensity level between an upper and lower heart-rate limit. Source: http://www.heartmonitors.com/exercisetips/heart_rate_basics.htm.) Since there are so many choices, it's important to consider which exercises are the most effective, especially if you have time restraints or special demands to meet, like wanting to be outside or not wanting to purchase a lot of equipment or join a gym.

There are no right or wrong cardio exercises. The best plan is simply to choose one or more that you enjoy. That way, you stand a better chance of sticking with it, and you will probably work harder.

Running is a great choice for a variety of reasons. It doesn't require special equipment (except for some good-quality shoes). You can run almost anywhere, anytime. It's high impact, which helps build strong bones and connective tissue. It gets your heart rate up more quickly than low-impact exercise. Last but not least, it helps you burn a lot of calories, especially when you crank it up by sprinting, incorporating interval training, or blasting into high gear by running up the occasional hill.

Cross-country skiing involves both the upper and lower body, and it doesn't take long for you to get your heart rate up to your target zone for optimal calorie burn.

Cycling, whether outdoors or on a machine, is also an effective cardio workout, and it is low impact. This is very important for people like me who have worn down the cartilage in their knees from too many squats over the years.

The elliptical trainer, next to the treadmill, is the most popular cardio machine at the gym. It allows your body to move smoothly in a natural way, without the impact of the treadmill. You can control the intensity by increasing resistance. You can go backward on an elliptical trainer, which is a little awkward at first, but it adds great variety and works your muscles in a different way.

Swimming is another great choice because, like cross-country skiing, it's a total body workout. The more body parts involved, the more calories you burn. Swimming is also extremely low impact, a plus for those with joint and other problems affected by impact.

The rowing machine offers physically demanding exercise for both the upper and lower body, which is wonderfully effective for maintaining a higher heart rate and burning calories. Like an elliptical trainer or stationary bike, different levels of resistance can be set, allowing you to get a challenging workout no matter what your fitness level.

Kickboxing is a good choice for exercisers who want to work hard with more choreographed workouts. Combining kicking and punching not only enhances your coordination and balance; it works both the upper and lower body, making this an excellent overall workout.

Walking, like running, is accessible: You don't need special equipment other than good walking shoes, it's low impact, and you can do it anywhere, anytime. It's harder to get your heart rate up with walking, but you can still get a good burn going, especially if you take in some hills. I walk at four-and-a-half miles an hour.

Does anyone jump rope anymore? This is another good calorie burner, with ropes being inexpensive and easy to transport.

Give your body a fighting chance to win

One of my exercises of choice is Tae Bo. Why? It's fast paced, there's a great deal of flexibility training for your core, it's intense and challenging, and there are no squats. Squats over the years have left me with knees that emit a high-pitched crunching sound. It's so loud that people look at me as if I need oiling. Not good!

The value of your cardio workout depends on two key components: the session length and the intensity. The harder you work the more calories you burn and the more fat you will lose. If you have a difficult time doing the math, most treadmills will provide an estimate of the calories you are potentially burning. When you get a chance, hop on the treadmill and experiment with how it feels when you walk at different speeds. Adjust the speed to allow you to burn the number of calories you want to burn, within your targeted session time. Test what that feels like, and push to work to that level when you engage in other cardio activity.

Here are some general cardio guidelines. For maximum fat loss, exercise thirty to sixty minutes per session. For maintenance and cardiovascular conditioning, exercise twenty to thirty minutes per session. Shoot for at least three sessions a week, and break a sweat! If you are not sweating, you are not working hard enough. As your fitness level improves, you will have to work harder to achieve the same gain.

If you want to really burn fat quickly, try seven sessions a week. It is a common perception that you exercise an hour after eating to burn off calories. In fact, a brisk walk or run outside or on the treadmill on an empty stomach every morning burns fat more efficiently and is a great way to start the day.

A compelling argument for exercising in the morning, every morning

Ninety percent of people who exercise regularly every morning stick it out over the long haul, even if they can only fit in ten or fifteen minutes. Morning exercise kick-starts your metabolism and keeps it functioning at a higher level for hours after you have worked out. Starting your day with any form of physical activity will loosen and limber up your body so you will feel alive and energized. Research shows that exercise increases mental acuity for an average of four to ten hours afterward.

Morning exercise reinforces a healthy mental mindset. So when it comes to making food choices, the tendency is to reach for more healthful foods. There is also a better comprehension of appetite and eating when you are hungry as opposed to simply because there is food around. Many people look at the morning workout as a time to look after and even pamper themselves, and often a missed day is regarded as a disappointment.

Morning exercise is easier to make a priority because the chaos of the day hasn't had a chance to jump the queue, causing you to reschedule or skip your workout.

With the right diet and cardio and four to six one-hour workout sessions a week, I am able to maintain my personal targeted body fat level. You can aim for a similar goal.

Several devices are available on the market to measure your maximum exertion capacity. Buy one to suit your preferred form of activity so you can comfortably push yourself to your physical limits but stay within your safe zone. You want to improve your health, not blow a gasket or drop dead.

Next up? Weight lifting for fat loss

If you don't want to lose your muscle while dieting for fat loss, you need to lift weights.

Weight training increases your lean body mass, which speeds up your metabolic rate so you can burn more calories at rest. This is your basal metabolic rate or BMR, which we calculated on the fifteenth hole. Your BMR is directly proportional to the amount of muscle you carry.

Of course, cardio burns fat during aerobic activity, making you actually leaner at the end of the session than when you began. Where weight lifting differs is that during the session, you are burning sugars. The primary fat-burning effect from weight training comes after the session from the increase in BMR and the increase in your post-exercise metabolic rate.

The best solution for targeting fat loss is a combination of cardio and lifting weights.

Here are some general weight-lifting guidelines. For maximum fat loss, work out thirty to sixty minutes per session. For example, for a training schedule of three sessions a week, a day on and a day off, do a full-body workout so your muscles can recover every other day. For daily training, alternate the muscles being worked. For instance, work your upper body on day one and your lower body on day two to allow for a day of rest and recovery in between sessions that use similar muscles. Try for at least three sessions a week, and break a sweat.

I don't ever want to be a fair-weather anything. Playing through the elements is always better than sitting on the sidelines

One of my No Excuses FIT Plan objectives outside of losing fat is to increase my club head speed for an improved golf swing. For this, I use Tae Bo to increase my core flexibility. I also use weight lifting to focus on my biceps, triceps, laterals, and abdominals to increase my upper-body strength. I think of the cardio portion of my sessions as the warm-up for my body, to reduce the risk of injury, and the weight lifting as building the power and strength I need.

There are lots of great magazines, books, and videos on the market to help you put together a fitness program that suits your requirements. I have just touched on the basics here. My main intention is to get you as psyched about creating and mastering your lifestyle prototype quest as I am about creating and mastering mine. The benefits of both weight lifting and cardio are well worth it. You'll feel strong, healthy, alive, and invigorated!

A stiff one

At the end of the week, I want to feel the effects of the exercise. That stiff feeling in my legs or shoulders or back reminds me that I have been working hard and, more importantly, that I am making progress. In winter, sometimes I'll take a walk around the lake in fresh snow with my heavy boots, or in summer I'll hike through the bush at the back of our house with leg and arm weights. It's a marvelous workout.

When it comes to cardio, I like to do a little bit of everything. Watching my fuel intake, I keep my exercise sessions as flexible as possible because I want to enjoy them. I want to achieve my goals, but I still want to have a life. A lot of my work life is creative but regimented, predictable, and predictably hectic. So I choose to look at exercise as an escape. I get to ditch details and deadlines for activity and, often, spontaneity. Ironically, I'm sometimes more stiffened from tension and stress at work than I am stiff and sore from working out.

It's important to remember that as soon as your muscles become accustomed to a certain level of weights and cardio, you'll no longer be stiff or sore. That means you are no longer building muscle, only maintaining your current level of muscle tone. You have to change up your regimen regularly if you want to continually build muscle and hit high on the stiffness meter. That's a challenge in itself!

The sanctity of the hum—call it meditation or call it getting zoned

Yes, the hum. It's that point where you shut everything around you off and focus, focus, focus.

As you exercise, you visualize intensely, and then there is a hush, then calm, then a light, soothing hum. The beat of your heart is the constant, a meditative rhythm, allowing you to move away from thinking in the moment, enabling you to get a real sense of who you are, every graceful movement, each repeating in succession and moving you closer to where you need to be.

There is something going on while we exercise. We feel it increasing with each day of working out. We gradually find what we have longed for—a higher level of personal reality, satisfaction, and gratification. We become increasingly aware of what we truly desire in life. We get zoned about what life will be like when we have achieved the feat of realizing our dreams. It is a peaceful state of complete, unadulterated mental and physical bliss, when all self-consciousness and self-doubt falls by the wayside and an overwhelming sense of clarity, of focus, and of our authentic self rejuvenates and percolates to the surface, rendering us a force to be dealt with. It pulls up from our toes and explodes out through our fingertips. It's a grandeur and brilliance taken to an exponential degree.

I first experienced this years ago while running. I would start out at an easy pace, then minor aches and pains would kick in, the odd stitch in my side. But I would persevere, and eventually all distraction would disappear, and I would hear only the beat of my heart as it seemed to synchronize with the melodic thud of my heavy-footed pace.

On purpose, with purpose

I am a "live in the moment" person. At the same time, I am highly focused. If I am in a social situation, joking around and having fun, I shut stresses and concern off. If I am golfing, I focus on my game, relaxing between plays. If I am in a situation where I can multitask effectively, I will, as this is a very familiar and comfortable state of mind for me.

On the other hand, there is a slightly out-of-focus state that I love to slip in and out of. If you have ever experienced a brilliant revelation while daydreaming or showering, you will know exactly what I am referring to.

It came to me in the shower!

Mindful power resting is that state of being where you are relaxed and calm, functioning on autopilot, so that unfinished ideas begin to register, formulate, and solidify.

Here is an exercise you can do to stimulate this process. Find a quiet private place in your house or even better, out of doors and lie on your back on a mat with a rolled towel positioned below your spine. Let your shoulders fall back gently. With your eyes shut, breathe in through your mouth, deeply and slowly, and exhale through your nose, and silently let yourself go.

When you are truly relaxed, powerful calmness encourages rest and mindful thought. The cloudiness and stress of the day dissipates, you are left with clear whole thoughts. You can regroup, rekindle, and regenerate. Mind and body acting as one: It is a harmonious balance.

When there is no distraction, there is clarity.

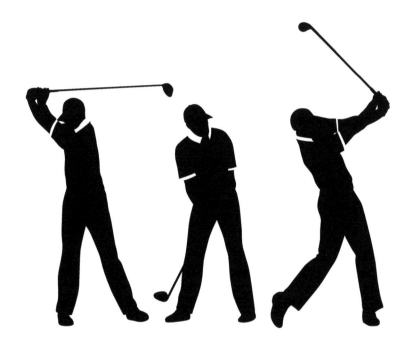

Visualize the Shot

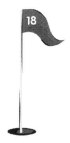

The 18th Hole – **Become a Champion**

I began the back nine by mentioning how I sometimes visualize myself in a practice swing, pulling back smoothly into my backswing and stopping. I then methodically run through a mental checklist to see whether I'm ready with the right grip, the right form, the right stance, and finally, whether I'm ready to take the shot. It's like a strategy opener, a recap and run through, mental and visual—what do I know and what am I going to tackle today?

So now, having completed the back nine, do you think you are ready for a fitness challenge? We have examined the key factors needed to visualize, strategize, and commit to acting and creating an effective lifestyle prototype. We have delved deep into the nature and importance of aspirations, expectations, motivation, and incentives. We have itemized what to consider when preparing to launch a new No Excuses FIT lifestyle, the reasons for doing so, and the results you may expect. And we have established a foundation for pushing our strategy into play and bridging all the valuable components from expectations and mindset to diet and exercise.

I recognize this may be tough for some people. Sometimes we can get overwhelmed, thinking it is too hard, too much work, or even too late for us. We may feel that too much time has elapsed between who we once were and who we have become and that our old, fitter, healthier self is irrecoverable. Yet we all have to start somewhere. Each of us has our own unique beginning, and if we dig deep enough, we know where to start. Now we just need to start!

It is not the thought that counts

It would be nice to be assured that we could glide along in perfect health without having to work at it, living a fabulous, carefree life without the threat of negative consequences. But unfortunately, that is not the case. We must all, individually and on a global level, take responsibility for our health and make it a priority.

The funny thing about life is that it seems to sneak up on you. Great intentions get set aside as you take care of business, whatever it is that needs your attention at that moment, and gradually the years pass. And you change, often so slowly that you don't recognize the changes, until one day while looking through old photos you think, "Wait! I have changed so much, I don't even look like me anymore!" That big change didn't just happen; you just suddenly woke up to it.

You need to look at health in the same way. Change occurs slowly, but that is all the more reason to pay attention. If you are oblivious to changes in your health, one day that ache or pain is going to mean something much more serious, and you are not going to like what you hear. Although change creeps up slowly, the phrase "life can turn on a dime" comes to mind.

It does happen. If you do not look after your health, it can take a sudden turn for the worse. And at that point, everything becomes real. It is like another old saying, "the straw that broke the camel's back." Change can occur suddenly, building to a crescendo and occurring abruptly after that one last straw is gently set in place, and you can be knocked to your knees. It takes an almost weightless straw to break the camel's proverbial back. The opportunity is lost for what you would have or could have done. The question becomes, "What do I do now?" but you'll find your answers are much more limited.

―――――

My take has always been to head off or prevent illness by taking the best possible care of my mental and physical health. I want to be in the best shape possible so, if necessary, I can fight the good fight if I do become ill. I believe my experience with having severe allergic reactions has prompted me to feel this way. I take life and health seriously.

Turn a potential life-or-death situation into a life-or-life situation

If your family has a history of illness, work to safeguard yourself against it by getting routine checkups and upgrading to a healthful lifestyle. Focus on preventing disease so you don't find yourself hoping that someone out there knows how to treat it. What it comes down to is deciding to champion a lifestyle committed to preserving your health.

Become a master Internet detective and learn all you can about your health. Believe that no one is as concerned about your health as you are—not your spouse, your best friend, or your doctor. Take on this responsibility for yourself. Have a physical and ask for a copy of the results. Alter your health and fitness program to yield improvement on your next physical. Consider which health risks, if any, hold potential threats for you, and then work to protect yourself.

Doctors are people too, and some are better than others. The bottom line: you and your doctor can arrive at better solutions if you come prepared with knowledge and informed, intelligent questions.

Question the automatic move to pharmaceuticals

When it comes to prescriptions, don't just accept them at face value. Ask specific, pointed questions and don't be shy. This is your health we're talking about. Ask: What exactly will this medication do for me? What are the probable side effects I should be aware of? What will happen if I don't take the medication? Are there alternative remedies? Is there anything you can do to improve your condition without the use of drugs? I don't like to sound negative here, but remember, every time a prescription is written, someone is getting paid. I am all for that. Just don't let it happen at the expense of your health.

Go from Band-Aids to bulletproof

It's up to you to now take the No Excuses FIT Lifestyle and use it as a lifestyle prototype. Be proactive about your life. Instead of smacking on another Band-Aid, do your best to become bulletproof.

I commend you for coming this far. Did you know that most people don't? They buy books and videos and gym memberships and nutritional supplements when they are in aspirational mode. They make the purchase, which makes them feel good, and they may feel good for a while, as long as they think they are still going to get around to the book, the video, or the gym. But they never actually make the transition from aspiration to action.

You, on the other hand, have invested the time and effort to study the life-changing material in this book. You have taken the first step, you know what to expect, and at this point, your expectations and motivation level are running high. I'm guessing you are anxious to improve your health and render yourself bulletproof against illness.

You now have knowledge, direction, a plan, and great expectations—of yourself and what you will achieve.

Fuel, energize, and rejuvenate

But you still have some work to do. I have not given you an exact diet but just an example of what I do, and I've given you an outline of how to create one for yourself in which you choose the foods you prefer. This is important because the more you make this lifestyle your own, the more likely you are to succeed. The only prerequisite is to stay within your daily budget of calories.

After you have your diet in place, buy yourself a two-month supply of multivitamins recommended for your sex and age group. There are many good-quality selections today. Twenty-five years ago, I had to take twenty-six pills a day to attain the same level of minerals and nutrients that I can get from six today. Most vitamin manufacturers today pay attention to the pill size as well, keeping them as small as possible so they are easier to swallow.

Mainstream health professionals, such as those in the American Medical Association, and many nutritionists, now recommend taking a multivitamin supplement every day. This is to ensure that everyone gets enough of these essential nutrients every day, even if your food choices are less than ideal. As well, it is often difficult for many of us to meet the ideal levels of daily mineral and nutrient requirements through the consumption of food alone, so take your multivitamins and think of them as insurance.

Hydrate, lubricate, oxygenate

To meet your daily water quota, check out the new breed of low-cal electrolyte replacement drink packets. The one I use has been designed specifically for rapid, healthful hydration and recovery. It is absorbed into the body significantly faster than water, allowing the body to replenish the electrolytes and minerals needed for rehydration. It also tastes good.

There are many products on the market that can increase hydration when added to water. Some claim an increase of eighty percent. If drinking water is difficult for you, you may want to seek out some of these products: Sqwincher Lite Qwik Stiks, Gatorade G2 Powder Sticks or Powerade Powder Sports Drink Concentrate.

Look for a combination of up to 80 grams of potassium, 45 grams of sodium, and up to 25 milligrams of magnesium, and try to keep the calories low.

You can also experiment and make your own electrolyte replacement drink. I use a packet of Crystal Light, eight ounces of water, 2 tbsp. of lemon juice, and a small pinch of salt.

Coconut is also a refreshing alternative for electrolyte replacement because it contains higher than average levels of potassium, one of the most important electrolytes for muscle function.

Flex, sculpt, and redefine

With regard to your cardio sessions, I again stress the value of doing what you enjoy. Try new things, keep it interesting, and change up your workout. One of the things I do to keep things fresh is to alternate between my old standby, the treadmill, and one of the non-gym exercise plans that come out in the monthly exercise magazines I buy. These creative workouts usually require the bare essentials such as lightweight free weights, a skip rope, a floor mat, or an exercise ball. Variety is important, and your body will benefit from exercising different muscle groups.

Weight lifting is the third corner of the health triangle that includes good nutrition and good cardio fitness. It's no secret that lifting weights has been my passion since I was in my late teens. A lean, well-rounded, toned, muscular yet sleek body is something to strive for, and it's especially gratifying when you can see and feel results quickly. This is especially true after a great workout when your muscles are taut and slightly swollen.

While I've given you some basic direction for putting your weight-lifting plan together, you should also choose a good instructional book or video to use as a guide or hire an experienced personal trainer to nail down the weights portion of your lifestyle.

A good practice is to use cardio as a fat burner and a warm-up for your weight program. When you are warmed up and loose from the cardio session, you have less risk of injury during the weights sessions.

Everything you do makes you better and stronger

For the best results, do the whole program in combination—a session with cardio followed by weights, done every other day to give your body a rest. Do three or four sessions a week for a minimum of ten weeks, but try to keep it going longer—perhaps a modified version. You may want to continue until you hit your target and then move into a modified program for maintenance.

Success is not random

Have you tried and failed to achieve your goals in the past? If so, I encourage you to think about this. Success is not random. Successful people are not just lucky. Success is developed over time from hard work and from a commitment to act and not give up. Remember what I said in the chapter called At the Turn? When you give up, you reward failure.

Create a plan, do a workout schedule to fit your weekday and weekend timetable, and don't break that pattern for your ten weeks. If you are going to take time off, plan it. Don't let your dreams run sideways. Haphazard actions don't bring results!

Doing a combination of cardio and weight training every other day for ten weeks doesn't mean you have to go to the gym. Start small. Along with a healthful eating plan, the following activities can get you started on your lifestyle prototype by providing a combination of cardio and impact (weight-bearing) exercise.

☞ Walk briskly to work in the morning.

☞ Go to the driving range at lunch.

☞ Throw a football with your kids before dinner.

☞ Take the dog for a one-mile fast walk after dinner.

☞ Do one hundred jumping jacks and grab a shower before bed.

Build your support team or become part of a support team

Need a little more inspiration? Get involved! Join a sports team or coach one. Look to others for assistance or become a mentor. Find a training buddy. Accept a local fitness challenge. Walk for the cure of your choice and encourage others to do the same. Build camaraderie in whatever you get involved in and watch your motivation jump to champion levels!

I wrote this book with the hope of inspiring you to take the action necessary for you to develop the body you've always wanted—and to take action immediately. Don't wait until tomorrow! I urge you to take what you've learned and begin now. Start with your next meal. Start working out today, if you're not doing so already. There is no need to put it off until New Year's, or after the holidays, or after the kids go back to school, or the first day of the month, or after final exams are over, or whenever—remember what brought you here. So please, don't wait. *No excuses!*

You only live once.
But if you live your life right,
once can mean everything!

You now have all the tools and information you need to begin working on a leaner, healthier, more muscular and attractive body today. You have learned:

o The importance of goal setting, how to set goals, and how to reach them.

o How to turn aspirations into expectations.

o Why diet alone won't provide the results you want and how to put a successful life-style prototype program together.

o Why body composition is more important than body weight.

o Why calories count and how to calculate your exact calorie requirements for losing fat as quickly as possible without going into starvation mode.

o The secrets of meal frequency and timing to get your metabolism racing at champion levels.

o The basics of what you need to know about protein, carbohydrates, and fat.

o How much water to drink to keep your energy levels high and your body burning fat efficiently and running at peak levels.

o How to construct you own meals and menu plans.

o The importance of taking a multivitamin as insurance.

o How much cardio you really need for maximum fat loss.

o Why weight training is critically important for fat loss.

o Why it's important for you to create your own plan as opposed to grabbing an off the shelf package. Your healthful lifestyle is yours to live, so it's important that you like what you are doing.

Okay, let's quickly recap the back nine:

The 10th Hole – Strategy Phase I: Auto-aspire: To effectively function in full auto-aspire mode, you need to open your mind and become intuitively aware of your thoughts and feelings, your authentic self—*not* the adult, always-in-control you that you present to the world day after day.

The 11th Hole – Strategy Phase II: Expectations and Being Proactive: When you begin to expect that there is always room for improvement, you put yourself in the driver's seat. Why wait for someone else to figure it out or do it? Expect that you are the one. Expect great outcomes. Expect that you are the best candidate and that you will achieve your goals.

The 12th Hole – Strategy Phase III: Motivation and Incentives: Most of us are continually engaged in some form of pursuit. We are seeking excellence within one or more areas in our lives, and that is the basis of our motivation. It is human nature to have a need to get ahead, need a little something more—it's in our DNA. Although we may not be certain of what we need at any given moment, we know there's something. It's a competitive itch and desire to improve that never goes away.

The 13th Hole – Strategy Phase IV: Visualization and Commitment: Visualization is a creative effort that can be developed and improved over time. You want to move from contemplating change to having a solid picture of change in your mind. You do that by strategically visualizing and then committing to act.

The 14th Hole – Strategy Phase V: Formulate a Curriculum: The simple task of taking a physical piece of paper and spilling words onto it can be a great beginning if you use it to detail your dreams, your quests, and your priorities. Add to it and upgrade it as you progress. Lists are a great form of visual aid.

The 15th Hole – Launch Your Success Action Plan: When you find something that works, and it works every time, why would you mess with it? We know that exercise works, and we know that a doctor-approved combination of vitamins and supplements works, so now let's consider what works when it comes to the consumption of food and how to lose fat. The answer? Counting calories. There are many ways to market and remarket this process, many very costly. However, we have a very simple solution here, a mathematical calculation for losing weight that works, and we know that it works every time!

The 16th Hole – The No Excuses FIT Lifestyle: The No Excuses FIT (Focused Intense Training) diet philosophy is a lifestyle prototype. It has evolved over the last thirty years. It is straightforward and simple, especially when you consider the reasons behind it. A healthful lifestyle evolves when you find the right combination of healthful eating habits and activity level that you can live with long term.

The 17th Hole – Exercise Your Options: It is much better to burn fat off than to diet it off. With exercise combined with proper nutrition, you can burn excess body fat, feed your muscles, and elevate your metabolism.

The 18th Hole – Become a Champion: I hope you feel eager to put all this knowledge to use and to reach your goals quickly, but don't be impatient. Give success a chance. There is nothing more rewarding than seeing and tracking your progress. Set expectations for yourself. Revel in your success each time you reach a small milestone. It is about the journey after all—your journey.

So, from your backswing, follow through, and hold the finish. I want to hear you say— *I did it!*

True sportsmanship is...

o *Knowing that you need your opponent because without him or her, there is no game*

o *Acknowledging that your opponent holds the same deep-rooted aspirations and expectations as you*

o *Knowing that, win or lose, you will walk off the course with pride*

o *Always taking the high road*

o *And always, always, always being a good sport*

True sportsmanship is excellence in motion!

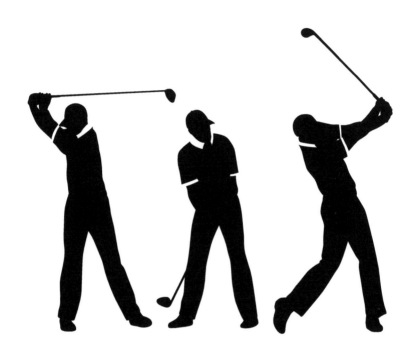

Play to Win

The 19ᵗʰ Hole:
Excellence in Motion

I love the concept of the nineteenth hole. It's the time after the game when you can chill out, when even the fiercest competitors let their guard down and relax. The nineteenth hole is also the fun after the game. It's grabbing a beer, having some laughs, and reliving the good shots. It's the time to look at your scorecard, see how you played, and formulate a game plan for what you will do differently the next time out. At that point, you dare to think that not only can you improve and excel, but you believe wholeheartedly that you will. It's a time for positive thinking.

When I think of excellence in motion, I think of the big picture. Because of the magnitude of this concept, I look at it from an aerial perspective. It is a mindset that challenges the boundaries of self-induced limits—that point where you aspire to exceed your expectations, where the mind-body-achievement connection resides and wins time and time again.

Our thoughts play a big role in all that we do in life. They guide us in our mental and physical strategies, how we feel about things, and how we will act. Positive progressive thoughts bring ideas to life and bring change to fruition. When we actively engage in the pursuit of excellence, questioning the relativity of the *impossible* and envisioning every last detail of the *possible,* we are set in motion.

Put some action on your good intentions

And now, it's almost time to put this book down and take action. Ask yourself honestly, *where do I go from here?* In a week, I'd like to you come back and answer the following questions:

o Have you written your No Excuses Success Action Plan?

o Have you created a working lifestyle proto-type and begun to work through it?

o Have you taken the fitness challenge in this book, and are you intent on *crushing* it?

o Have you taken the other challenges I've provided in this book to heart?

It has been my objective to help you learn how to say no to everyday excuses so you can build an authentic lifestyle prototype. It is important to understand the value of the continual search for excellence and the need to create a strong mind, a sleek physique, and optimal health for yourself. When you do that, you will fully appreciate and experience the feeling of being a champion in all areas of your life. You will have created your own excellence in motion.

Our bodies are more than just a vehicle for our minds. They are the inspiration!

It is the combination of the mind, the body, and the spirit working together—the mind-body-achievement connection—that is the basis of a lifestyle prototype of excellence. The three work together toward the goal of making you a champion in any areas of your life that you desire to be. And healthy competition and good sportsmanship in any sport or, in a broader sense, in any area of your personal or professional life, should also be embraced as key elements to success.

It's not enough to fill your head with wondrous ideas—you must initiate action

Life's best mentors and coaches are those who believe in you and your potential, sometimes even before you do. When the coach you have strived to impress slaps you on the back and says, "I knew you could do it!" with pride and respect, memorize that moment! Not only have you earned it, but keeping that sense of accomplishment alive in your mind will help you to visualize and to focus on achieving your next goal, and the one after that.

Most golfers work hard to improve their game by taking action. It's important to practice all the tough shots repeatedly in order to master them, and you need to record everything on your scorecard so you know your strengths and weaknesses. As much as there are days when you will wonder what you're doing on the course, there are others when you can do no wrong. It is the pro-like shots that keep you coming back, no matter how few and far between they may be. It is that spark of excellence, where everything you have diligently worked for comes together, that point where it is all worthwhile.

Excellence prospers in the absence of excuses

Our minds are always on alert, ready to serve and protect us, to help us survive threats (whether real or imagined) and to define our perception of our role in life. The *No Excuses* mind is even more sharply aligned; trained to operate strategically on a higher level and to tap into your ability to achieve your highest potential. The lessons of being limitless, taking an aerial perspective, identifying aspirations, managing excuses, pushing yourself past preconceived limits, finding your self-motivation, inspiration, and incentive, in conjunction with developing a vision of what is possible are all part of building a master life strategy.

Now armed with Fit Mind–Fit Body strategies, you are ready to build a focused and highly productive life—to define your own *excellence in motion*.

**Explore, experience, evolve,
and exceed your expectations!
No Excuses!**

Glossary of Golf Terms

A

"A" position – The "A" position is that position which allows the best approach for your next shot.

Address – (n., adj.) Address refers to the golfer's position when preparing to make a stroke (hit the ball).

Address the ball – (v.) Addressing the ball means you are in position and prepared to hit the ball. At this point, your main concern is whether you are properly aimed at your intended target and whether you are ready to take your shot.

Alignment – Alignment refers to the direction of the body and club when in the address position— for example, when you line up your body drawing a swing direction parallel to the target with your clubface square to the target.

Approach shot – The approach shot is a shot where your intended target is the green.

At the turn – At the turn traditionally refers to having completed the first nine holes of golf and getting ready for the back nine or last set of nine holes to be played.

B

Back nine – The last nine holes (ten to eighteen) of an eighteen-hole golf course.

Ball position – Ball position is the position of the ball relative to a player's stance and the target at address. The ball is considered to be *forward* in the players' stance if the ball is nearer the front foot or *back* in the player's stance if the ball is closer to the rear foot as relative to the target.

Best ball – Best ball is a match where an individual plays against the better ball of two, or the best ball of three.

Birdie – A birdie is a score of one under (less than) par for a hole.

Bunker – A bunker is a hollow or valley of some kind, usually filled with sand. A bunker is also known as a trap or sand trap.

C

Chip – A chip is a shot played from around the green, usually played with a pitching wedge or a sand wedge.

Course management – Course management or game management is the use of strategy to emphasize strengths and compensate for weaknesses in order for the player to make his or her way around the golf course as efficiently and effectively as possible.

D

Driver – The driver is also known as the 1 wood. It is the most powerful club in the set and used to achieve maximum distance from the tee.

Driving range – A driving range is an area, separate from the golf course, designated for hitting practice balls.

E

Errant shot – An errant shot is one that leaves you in long grass, under a tree, in loose, tangled brush, or in the water.

F

Fairway – The fairway is the closely mown proper route between the tee and the green.

Fairway woods – Fairway woods 2, 3, 4, 5, and sometimes higher-numbered woods are designed for use when the ball is in play after the tee shot. These clubs are often referred to as fairway metals today, as they are more commonly made of metal rather than wood.

Fringe – The fringe is the collar of slightly longer grass around the closely mown putting surface of the green.

Front nine – The front nine or front denotes the first nine holes (one to nine) of an eighteen-hole golf course.

G

Green – The green is the most closely mown and smooth area of the course, which is specifically prepared for putting. The green is also referred to as the putting green, putting surface, and the dance floor. When you are on the green, you're dancing!

Golf course – A golf course consists of a series of holes, usually two sets of nine, where each hole consists of a teeing ground, fairway, rough, and other hazards, and a green with a flag or pin, and cup, all designed for the game of golf.

Grip – A grip is the handle of a golf club, usually covered with rubber or leather. Alternatively, a player's grip refers to the method of holding a golf club properly.

H

Handicap – A handicap is the average difference between a series of a player's scores and a set standard.

Hazard – A hazard is any bunker (a hollow or valley of some kind, usually filled with sand) or water hazard (ocean, lake, pond, river, ditch, etc., usually marked with either white or red stakes or lines), even a sloped bank, that can hinder you from making par.

Hole – The hole, 4-¼" in diameter, into which the golf ball is played.

Hole-in-one – A hole-in-one is a score of one on a hole. The perfect shot!

I

In play – In play officially refers to when the ball is hit from the tee and comes to rest anywhere on the course, not out of bounds. Informally, a ball that is in play is playable.

Iron – An iron is a club with a head made of steel or iron with a relatively narrow sole (footprint), with varying lofts, and numbered one through nine, including a variety of wedges. That being said, the most common array of irons carried in a set of golf clubs is the 3 iron through pitching wedge. Many golfers add a sand wedge to the mix and/or a 1 or 2 iron, a gap wedge, or a lob wedge.

L

Leader board – A leader board is a scoreboard showing the top performers in a golf tournament or competition.

Lie – The lie is the position in which the golf ball comes to rest.

Loft – The loft is the angle of the club head relative to the shaft of the club from the frontal plane. Loft produces more or less height and makes the ball rise.

Lost ball – A golf ball is considered to be lost if after a five-minute search, it cannot be found. The player is penalized one stroke.

M

Match play – A match play is a game of golf in which you compete on a hole-by-hole basis.

Mishit – A mishit is any stroke that is not shot solidly.

Mulligan – A mulligan or mullie is a do-over. A player takes a second attempt or replay of a shot when he doesn't like the result of the first.

Muscle memory – Muscle memory is a phrase referring to the nervous system's ability to memorize, or automatically reproduce, a motion with which the muscles have become familiar.

N

Nineteenth hole – The nineteenth hole (or 19th hole) is the bar or lounge after the round of golf.

O

Out of bounds – Out of bounds or OB is an area that is not part of the course and on which play is not permitted. White stakes usually mark the out-of-bounds area.

P

Par – Par is the standard number of strokes in which a scratch golfer, a golfer with a zero handicap, is expected to complete a hole.

Par for the course – Par for the course is the standard number of strokes in which a scratch golfer, a golfer with a zero handicap, is expected to complete eighteen holes.

Penalty stroke – A penalty stroke is a stroke added to the player's score for a variety of reasons such as a lost ball or an unplayable lie, in accordance with the rules of golf.

Pitch – A pitch or pitch shot is a relatively short, lofted shot designed to land softly and without a lot of roll.

Pitching wedge – A pitching wedge, P, PW, or W is a lofted short iron.

Practice green – See green.

Practice range – See driving range.

Pre-shot routine – A pre-shot or pre-swing routine is a procedure or consistent sequence used as preparation prior to hitting a golf shot. There are three basic considerations to keep in mind: 1) Am

I properly set up? 2) Am I properly aligned? 3) Is my ball in the correct position? You need to take a minute to visualize the shot from behind the ball and perhaps even choose an intermediate spot in front of the ball, in line with your primary target, to use as an alignment aid.

Putt – A putt is a shot generally hit with a putter that is intended to make a ball roll on or from just off the putting green.

Putter – A putter is a club with a fairly straight face and very little loft used for putting.

Putting green – See green.

R

Range – See driving range.

Recovery shot – A recovery shot is a shot that will set up the succeeding shot—a shot that has a good lie so that you are in position to make your next shot. A recovery shot is played to extricate oneself from trouble after an errant shot.

Recreational golfer – A recreational golfer is an amateur player who plays for recreation or fun and, therefore, uses a more relaxed interpretation of the rules of golf.

Regulation – Regulation or being on the green in regulation, means playing your ball onto the green in the prescribed number of strokes as determined by par or simply par for the hole, less two strokes for putting.

Round – A round or round of golf is eighteen holes, broken up into two sets of nine.

Rough – The rough is the area of less kempt grass and vegetation bordering the fairway. Playing from the rough generally entails more difficulty in making clean contact with the ball.

Rule #27 – Ball lost or out of bounds. This rule states that if you lose a ball hit from the tee, you can hit from the tee again or drop a ball two club-lengths back from where your ball exited the fairway. Either way, your score is one stroke from the tee plus one penalty stroke for the lost ball. In other words, you are now hitting three—one stroke for the lost shot plus the other two from the tee, thus the term "three off the tee."

S

Sand Trap – See bunker.

Sand wedge – A sand wedge, sandwedge, or sand iron is a lofted club with a flange specifically designed for use in the sand.

Sandbagger – Sandbagger is a euphemism for a liar or cheater. This refers to a golfer who lies about his or her ability in order to gain advantage over opponents in a match or wager game.

Score – A score is the number of strokes taken on a hole or course.

Scorecard – A scorecard or card is a preprinted card usually provided by the golf course, used to record and tally scores during and after a round of golf.

Scratch – Scratch is a zero handicap.

Scratch player – A scratch player is one who is expected to play the course in par.

Set of clubs – A set of clubs includes a maximum of fourteen—usually four woods, nine irons, and one putter.

Setup – see address.

Short game – The short game in golf refers to approach shots to the green and putting. Some people think of the short game as anything inside of one hundred yards, and others think of it as a shot on or in the immediate vicinity of the green.

Shot – A shot or stroke in golf refers to both the act of swinging a club with the intention of striking the ball (n.) and the past tense of striking the ball (v.).

Shot planner – See pre-shot routine.

Skins – Skins is a hole-by-hole competition or wager in which the lowest score wins. When there is a tie, the win carries over to the next hole until there is finally a lowest score.

Slice – A slice or banana ball is a faulty shot that curves left to right in the air (for a right-handed player).

Slope – The slope of a golf course is a rating of the relative playing difficulty of a course for players who are not scratch golfers.

Stance – Stance is the player's position when the feet are set, in alignment, ready to play the ball.

Straight up – Playing a game of golf straight up refers to playing a competition or wager where no handicap is used to adjust the players' scores.

Stroke – See shot.

Stroke play – Stroke play is a game of golf where you compete against others based on your total score for eighteen holes.

Swing – A golf swing is the player's physical motion used to make a stroke.

Swing thought – A swing thought is a short catch phrase intended to help the player keep his or her mind in the game and focused on making the shot.

T

Target – A target is the location where you intend a shot ball to lie or finish.

Tee – The tee is the flat, sometimes raised, area from which first shots at each hole are played, as well as a small device used to set the ball up above the ground in preparation for taking a shot.

Tee shot – A tee shot is the first shot on a hole where the ball was shot off a tee.

Three off the tee – If a ball hit from the tee is lost, out of bounds, or unplayable, the player is penalized one stroke and then tees off again. The score is one stroke from the tee plus one penalty stroke for the lost ball, and now you are hitting a third shot.

Trap – See bunker.

Trust your swing – A phrase meaning that when you trust your swing, you are confident in your ability to make solid and clean contact with the ball.

V

Visualize the shot – When you visualize the shot you are able to use mental imagery to see the shot required.

W

Water hazard – A water hazard is any sea, lake, or pond, whether it contains water or not, usually marked with either yellow or red stakes or lines.

Wedge – A wedge is a subset of irons, shorter in length, with significant loft and generally used in short game play. There are various wedges include the pitching wedge, sand wedge, lob wedge, third wedge, and utility wedge.

Wood – See driver and fairway woods.

Work the ball – To work the ball means to deliberately shape or curve a shot to your advantage.

Note to the Reader

Watch for the next book in the *3 Off the Tee* series of motivational self-improvement books.

About the Author

Lorii Myers is an empowered employee turned entrepreneur. Her three-plus decades of business experience include a wide variety of career challenges: business manager, controller, senior management member, business owner, and award-winning author.

Myers believes that we should aspire to learn from those who inspire us, and she was therefore careful to choose her early employment opportunities well. She worked for entrepreneurial companies that were owned or managed by formidable entrepreneurs. When asked what she learned, Myers is quick with the answer—"The right attitude is everything!"

In her early thirties, Myers left the security of employment to fulfill her own entrepreneurial aspirations. Because of her personal quest to explore every opportunity life offers, she brings a wealth of knowledge and experience to this book.

Please feel free to contact the author and share your successes:

Lorii@3-Off-the-Tee.com

Other books by Lorii Myers:

3 Off the Tee: Targeting Success

3 Off the Tee: Make it Happen

21147766R00177

Made in the USA
Charleston, SC
09 August 2013